T0226406

Current Management of Pancreatic Cancer

Editors

SUSAN TSAI
DOUGLAS B. EVANS

SURGICAL ONCOLOGY CLINICS OF NORTH AMERICA

www.surgonc.theclinics.com

Consulting Editor
TIMOTHY M. PAWLIK

October 2021 • Volume 30 • Number 4

ELSEVIER

1600 John F. Kennedy Boulevard • Suite 1800 • Philadelphia, Pennsylvania, 19103-2899

http://www.theclinics.com

SURGICAL ONCOLOGY CLINICS OF NORTH AMERICA Volume 30, Number 4
October 2021 ISSN 1055-3207, ISBN-13: 978-0-323-81359-4

Editor: John Vassallo (j.vassallo@elsevier.com)
Developmental Editor: Diana Ang

Surgical Oncology Clinics of North America (ISSN 1055-3207) is published quarterly by Elsevier Inc., 360 Park Avenue South, New York, NY 10010-1710. Months of publication are January, April, July, and October. Business and Editorial Offices: 1600 John F. Kennedy Blvd., Ste. 1800, Philadelphia, PA 19103-2899. Customer Service Office: 3251 Riverport Lane, Maryland Heights, MO 63043. Periodicals postage paid at New York, NY and additional mailing offices. Subscription prices are $315.00 per year (US individuals), $750.00 (US institutions) $100.00 (US student/resident), $352.00 (Canadian individuals), $784.00 (Canadian institutions), $100.00 (Canadian student/resident), $456.00 (foreign individuals), $784.00 (foreign institutions), and $205.00 (foreign student/resident). Foreign air speed delivery is included in all *Clinics* subscription prices. All prices are subject to change without notice. **POSTMASTER**: Send address changes to *Surgical Oncology Clinics of North America*, Elsevier Health Science Division, Subscription Customer Service, 3251 Riverport Lane, Maryland Heights, MO 63043. **Customer Service: 1-800-654-2452 (US and Canada). 314-447-8871 (outside US and Canada). Fax: 314-447-8029. E-mail: journalscustomerservice-usa@elsevier.com (for print support); journalsonline support-usa@elsevier.com (for online support).**

Reprints. For copies of 100 or more, of articles in this publication, please contact the Commercial Reprints Department, Elsevier Inc., 360 Park Avenue South, New York, New York 10010-1710. Tel. 212-633-3874; Fax: 212-633-3820; E-mail: reprints@elsevier.com.

Surgical Oncology Clinics of North America is covered in *MEDLINE/PubMed (Index Medicus)* and *EMBASE/ Excerpta Medica, Current Contents/Clinical Medicine, and ISI/BIOMED.*

Contributors

CONSULTING EDITOR

TIMOTHY M. PAWLIK, MD, MPH, MTS, PhD, FACS, FRACS (Hon.)
Professor and Chair, Department of Surgery, The Urban Meyer III and Shelley Meyer Chair for Cancer Research, Professor of Surgery, Oncology, Health Services Management and Policy, Surgeon in Chief, The Ohio State University Wexner Medical Center, Columbus, Ohio, USA

EDITORS

SUSAN TSAI, MD, MHS
Director, LaBahn Pancreatic Cancer Program, Medical College of Wisconsin, Milwaukee, Wisconsin, USA

DOUGLAS B. EVANS, MD
Professor and Chair, Department of Surgery, Medical College of Wisconsin, Milwaukee, Wisconsin, USA

AUTHORS

VOLKAN ADSAY, MD
Professor, Head of Surgical Sciences Department, Chair, Department of Pathology, Koc University School of Medicine and KUTTAM Research Center, Koc University Hospital, Istanbul, Turkey

LEAH H. BILLER, MD
Department of Medical Oncology, Dana-Farber Cancer Institute, Harvard Medical School, Boston, Massachusetts, USA

SAKTI CHAKRABARTI, MD
Associate Professor, Division of Hematology and Oncology, Department of Medicine, LaBahn Pancreatic Cancer Program, Medical College of Wisconsin, Milwaukee, Wisconsin, USA

KENNETH J. CHANG, MD
Division of Gastroenterology and Hepatology, Digestive Health Institute, University of California, Irvine, Orange, California, USA

KATHLEEN K. CHRISTIANS, MD
Professor, Department of Surgery, Medical College of Wisconsin, Milwaukee, Wisconsin, USA

CHRISTOPHER H. CRANE, MD
Department of Radiation Oncology, Memorial Sloan Kettering Cancer Center, New York, New York, USA

KULWINDER S. DUA, MD, DMSc, FRCP (L), FRCP (E), FACP, MASGE
Division of Gastroenterology and Hepatology, Medical College of Wisconsin, Milwaukee, Wisconsin, USA

BETH ERICKSON, MD
Departments of Radiation Oncology and Surgery, Froedtert & the Medical College of Wisconsin, Milwaukee, Wisconsin, USA

DOUGLAS B. EVANS, MD
Professor and Chair, Department of Surgery, Medical College of Wisconsin, Milwaukee, Wisconsin, USA

MONA FOTH, PhD
Huntsman Cancer Institute, University of Utah, Salt Lake City, Utah, USA

IGNACIO GARRIDO-LAGUNA, MD, PhD
Huntsman Cancer Institute, University of Utah, Department of Internal Medicine, Division of Oncology, University of Utah School of Medicine, Salt Lake City, Utah, USA

BEN GEORGE, MD
William F. Stapp Endowed Chair, Medical Director, Clinical Trials Office, Associate Professor of Medicine, Mary Ann and Charles LaBahn Pancreatic Cancer Program, Division of Hematology and Oncology, Medical College of Wisconsin, Milwaukee, Wisconsin, USA

MICHAEL GOGGINS, MB, MD
Professor of Pathology, Medicine and Oncology, Johns Hopkins University, Baltimore, Maryland, USA

MICHAEL O. GRIFFIN, MD, PhD
Associate Professor, Departments of Radiology and Surgery, Medical College of Wisconsin, Milwaukee, Wisconsin, USA

WILLIAM A. HALL, MD
Departments of Radiation Oncology and Surgery, Froedtert & the Medical College of Wisconsin, Graduate School of Biomedical Sciences, Medical College of Wisconsin, Milwaukee, Wisconsin, USA

MANDANA KAMGAR, MD, MPH
Assistant Professor, Division of Hematology and Oncology, Department of Medicine, LaBahn Pancreatic Cancer Program, Medical College of Wisconsin, Milwaukee, Wisconsin, USA

JOSEPH F. KEARNEY, MD
Resident, Surgery, The University of North Carolina at Chapel Hill, Chapel Hill, North Carolina, USA

CONAN G. KINSEY, MD, PhD
Huntsman Cancer Institute, University of Utah, Department of Internal Medicine, Division of Oncology, University of Utah School of Medicine, Salt Lake City, Utah, USA

MARTIN MCKINNEY, MD
Assistant Professor, Department of Radiology, Medical College of Wisconsin, Milwaukee, Wisconsin, USA

A. JAMES MOSER, MD
Professor of Surgery, Harvard Medical School, Co-Director, Pancreas and Liver Institute, Beth Israel Deaconess Medical Canter, Boston, Massachusetts, USA

YOUSUKE NAKAI, MD
Department of Endoscopy and Endoscopic Surgery, The University of Tokyo Hospital, Tokyo, Japan

IBRAHIM NASSOUR, MD, MSCS
Surgical Oncology Fellow, University of Pittsburgh Medical Center, Pittsburgh, Pennsylvania, USA

ALESSANDRO PANICCIA, MD
Assistant Professor of Surgery, University of Pittsburgh Medical Center, Pittsburgh, Pennsylvania, USA

MARIANNA V. PAPAGEORGE, MD
Department of Surgery, Boston Medical Center, Boston University School of Medicine, Boston, Massachusetts, USA

ADITYA SHREENIVAS, MD, MS
Assistant Professor, Division of Hematology and Oncology, Department of Medicine, LaBahn Pancreatic Cancer Program, Medical College of Wisconsin, Milwaukee, Wisconsin, USA

ZACHARY SMITH, MD
Division of Gastroenterology and Hepatology, Medical College of Wisconsin, Milwaukee, Wisconsin, USA

PARAG P. TOLAT, MD
Associate Professor, Departments of Radiology and Surgery, Medical College of Wisconsin, Milwaukee, Wisconsin, USA

SUSAN TSAI, MD, MHS
Director, LaBahn Pancreatic Cancer Program, Medical College of Wisconsin, Milwaukee, Wisconsin, USA

JENNIFER F. TSENG, MD, MPH
James Utley Professor and Chair, Department of Surgery, Boston Medical Center, Boston University School of Medicine, Boston, Massachusetts, USA

ERIN P. WARD, MD
Surgical Oncology Division, Department of Surgery, Medical College of Wisconsin, Milwaukee, Wisconsin, USA

BRIAN M. WOLPIN, MD, MPH
Department of Medical Oncology, Dana-Farber Cancer Institute, Harvard Medical School, Boston, Massachusetts, USA

JEN JEN YEH, MD
Professor, Surgery and Pharmacology, The University of North Carolina at Chapel Hill, Chapel Hill, North Carolina, USA

HERBERT J. ZEH, III, MD
Professor and Chair, Department of Surgery, UT Southwestern (University of Texas), Dallas, Texas, USA

AMER H. ZUREIKAT, MD, FACS
Associate Professor of Surgery, Chief, Division of Surgical Oncology, University of Pittsburgh Medical Center, Pittsburgh, Pennsylvania, USA

Contents

Foreword: Pancreatic Cancer   xiii

Timothy M. Pawlik

Preface: Updates on the Management of Pancreatic Cancer   xvii

Susan Tsai and Douglas B. Evans

Pathology and Molecular Characteristics of Pancreatic Cancer   609

Joseph F. Kearney, Volkan Adsay, and Jen Jen Yeh

> Pancreatic ductal adenocarcinoma (PDAC) is the most common type of pancreatic cancer. However, it should be kept in mind that there are other pancreatic cancers that are classified by their cellular lineage: acinar cell carcinomas (acinar differentiation), neuroendocrine neoplasms (arising from the islets), solid-pseudopapillary neoplasms (showing no discernible cell lineage), and pancreatoblastomas (characterized by multiphenotypic differentiation, including acinar endocrine and ductal). This article focuses on the molecular and pathology alterations in PDAC.

Multimodality Imaging for the Staging of Pancreatic Cancer   621

Martin McKinney, Michael O. Griffin, and Parag P. Tolat

> Imaging plays a key role in the diagnosis, staging, and follow-up of pancreatic ductal adenocarcinoma. The pancreatic protocol dual-phase multidetector computed tomography scan is the imaging modality of choice. A computed tomography scan is highly accurate for pancreatic tumor detection, assessment of resectability, and detection of metastatic disease. This article reviews key principles of the acquisition, interpretation, and reporting of pancreatic ductal adenocarcinoma imaging with computed tomography scanning and highlights potential roles for newer and supplemental imaging technologies. We discuss the importance of structured interpretation and reporting for providing the most complete and accurate assessment of tumor stage and resectability.

Advanced Endoscopic Techniques for the Diagnosis of Pancreatic Cancer and Management of Biliary and GastricOutlet Obstruction   639

Yousuke Nakai, Zachary Smith, Kenneth J. Chang, and Kulwinder S. Dua

> Following high-quality imaging studies for staging, endoscopic ultrasound examination fine needle aspiration/biopsy is the preferred modality for tissue diagnosis of pancreatic cancer. Endoscopic retrograde cholangiopancreatography with metal stent placement is used for palliation of malignant biliary obstruction. Metal stents can be placed in patients with resectable pancreatic cancer in whom surgery is going to be delayed. For palliation of gastric outlet obstruction,

endoscopic enteral stenting is often selected because of its less invasiveness. Endoscopic ultrasound-guided biliary drainage for malignant biliary obstruction or gastrojejunostomy for gastric outlet obstruction are emerging less invasive techniques as compared with palliative surgery.

Current Controversies in Neoadjuvant Therapy for Pancreatic Cancer   657

Erin P. Ward, Herbert J. Zeh III, and Susan Tsai

Over the last several decades, there have been significant changes in the management of patients with localized pancreatic cancer. The rationale for an evolution toward a neoadjuvant approach and summary of relevant clinical trials is reviewed. Controversies in identifying optimal neoadjuvant therapeutic approaches are discussed.

Evolution of Systemic Therapy in Metastatic Pancreatic Ductal Adenocarcinoma   673

Mandana Kamgar, Sakti Chakrabarti, Aditya Shreenivas, and Ben George

Pancreatic ductal adenocarcinoma is characterized by early systemic dissemination, a complex tumor microenvironment, as well as significant intratumoral and intertumoral heterogeneity. Treatment options and survival in pancreatic ductal adenocarcinoma have improved steadily over the last 3 decades. Although cytotoxic chemotherapy is currently the mainstay of treatment for pancreatic ductal adenocarcinoma, evolving therapeutic strategies are aimed at targeting the tumor microenvironment, metabolism, and the tumor–host immune balance.

Precision Medicine and Pancreatic Cancer   693

Ben George

For several decades, cytotoxic chemotherapy was the mainstay of treatment for pancreatic ductal adenocarcinoma (PDAC). Advances in molecular profiling have identified predictive genomic alterations in PDAC—the germline and somatic genome are now routinely interrogated in patients with PDAC because of their therapeutic relevance. The composite role of the epithelial cell compartment and the tumor microenvironment in defining PDAC biology needs further elucidation to deconvolute the spatiotemporal heterogeneity appreciated in this disease. Novel clinical trial approaches leveraging signal seeking, adaptive statistical designs, and master protocols using several candidate drugs that target relevant therapeutic targets are essential to unlocking the potential of precision medicine in PDAC.

Therapeutic Targeting of Autophagy in Pancreatic Cancer   709

Mona Foth, Ignacio Garrido-Laguna, and Conan G. Kinsey

This article provides a brief review of the therapeutic opportunity of inhibiting autophagy in pancreatic cancer. The autophagic process, importance of autophagy in pancreatic cancer, relevant clinical trials, and new agents in preclinical and clinical development are discussed.

Evolving Concepts Regarding Radiation Therapy for Pancreatic Cancer   719

William A. Hall, Beth Erickson, and Christopher H. Crane

In todays practice most institutions individualize the use of adjuvant, neo-adjuvant, and definitive RT based on their interpretation of the available data. This review highlights novel concepts and approaches to the use of RT that should be considered by the surgical oncologist.

Pancreaticoduodenectomy and Vascular Reconstruction: Indications and Techniques   731

Kathleen K. Christians and Douglas B. Evans

Pancreaticoduodenectomy with vascular resection/reconstruction can be safely completed following 6 standard steps plus basic principles of vascular surgery. Particular attention is paid to the location of the tumor relative to the 2 first-order vein branches, portal vein —splenic vein–superior mesenteric vein confluence, inferior mesenteric vein, and the presence of arterial perineural invasion. Successful resection following neoadjuvant therapy can result in median survival 3 times that of historical controls.

Minimally Invasive Techniques for Pancreatic Resection   747

Ibrahim Nassour, Alessandro Paniccia, A. James Moser, and Amer H. Zureikat

There is increasing interest in the role of minimally invasive surgery (MIS) for pancreatectomy. Prospective data indicate significant advantages for MIS when performed for left-sided pancreatic pathologies and may be deemed as the standard of care. However, there is reluctance in implementing this technique to pancreaticoduodenectomy because of the complexity of the operation and the mixed results from randomized trials. A detailed description of the technical aspects of robotic pancreaticoduodenectomy and distal pancreatectomy is presented in this article in addition to a summary of the most important prospective and cohort studies. We also provide insights into patient selection and the learning curve of MIS surgery for pancreatectomy.

Health Care Disparities and the Future of Pancreatic Cancer Care   759

Marianna V. Papageorge, Douglas B. Evans, and Jennifer F. Tseng

There have been tremendous advances in the diagnosis and treatment of pancreatic cancer in the past decade, yet we are failing to achieve equitable outcomes for all patient populations. Disparities exist in the incidence, diagnosis, treatment, and outcomes of patients with pancreatic cancer. Inequities are based on racial and ethnic group, sex, socioeconomic status, and geography. To address disparities, future steps must focus on research methods, including collection and methodology, and policy measures, including access, patient tools, hospital incentives, and workforce diversity. Through these comprehensive efforts, we can begin to rectify inequitable care for treatment of patients with pancreatic cancer.

Inherited Pancreatic Cancer Syndromes and High-Risk Screening   773

Leah H. Biller, Brian M. Wolpin, and Michael Goggins

Pancreatic cancer is the third leading cause of cancer death in the United States, with a 5-year survival rate of 9%. Individuals with inherited pancreatic cancer syndromes are at an increased risk for developing pancreatic cancer and may benefit from pancreatic cancer surveillance with the goal to detect and intervene on early-stage cancer or high-risk precursor lesions. Given the screening implications for family members and therapeutic implications for probands, all patients diagnosed with pancreatic cancer are recommended to undergo germline genetic testing.

SURGICAL ONCOLOGY
CLINICS OF NORTH AMERICA

FORTHCOMING ISSUES

January 2022
Disparities and Determinants of Health in Surgical Oncology
Oluwadamilola "Lola" Fayanju, *Editor*

April 2022
Colorectal Cancer
Traci L. Hedrick, *Editor*

July 2022
Sarcoma
Chandrajit P. Raut and Alessandro Gronchi, *Editors*

RECENT ISSUES

July 2021
Palliative Care in Surgical Oncology
Bridget N. Fahy, *Editor*

April 2021
Pediatric Cancer
Roshni Dasgupta, *Editor*

January 2021
Management of Metastatic Liver Tumors
Michael D'Angelica, *Editor*

Foreword
Pancreatic Cancer

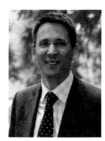

Timothy M. Pawlik, MD, MPH, MTS, PhD, FACS, FRACS (Hon.)
Consulting Editor

This issue of the *Surgical Oncology Clinics of North America* focuses on the management of pancreatic cancer. Pancreatic cancer is the seventh leading cause of cancer-related deaths worldwide with over 430,000 related deaths annually.[1] Unlike some other cancers, the incidence of pancreatic cancer continues to increase with relatively little improvement in survival. Despite some advances over the last several decades, pancreatic cancer has been characterized by tumor cell resistance to chemotherapy agents, which has resulted in the failure of many traditional cancer treatments. In addition, surgical resection, which offers the only chance of cure for pancreatic cancer, is only feasible in roughly 15% to 20% of cases at the time of presentation. Resectability may be limited due to involvement/abutment of the tumor with major vessels, such as the portal vein/superior mesenteric vein or the hepatic/superior mesenteric artery. Recent data provide insight into the earliest events of cellular invasion in situ and suggest that inflammation enhances cancer progression in part by facilitating epithelial-to-mesenchymal behavior with early dissemination of disease.[2] In turn, most data would suggest that pancreatic cancer is a systemic disease at the time of presentation even among many patients with early-stage tumors. As such, there has been broad adoption of neoadjuvant strategies for locally advanced, unresectable, or "borderline" resectable pancreatic cancer; in addition, neoadjuvant systemic therapy is widely used even in the setting of early-stage disease that may be technically resectable on presentation. While systemic chemotherapy was traditionally largely ineffective, the introduction of FOLFIRINOX (oxaliplatin plus irinotecan with leucovorin and short-term infusional fluorouracil) has improved efficacy and has a demonstrated survival benefit compared with gemcitabine monotherapy.[3] Other recent systemic options include gemcitabine with abraxane, as well as molecularly based targeted agents. Advances in locoregional therapy, including intraoperative radiotherapy, as well as stereotactic beam radiotherapy have also been utilized with varying success. Advances

Surg Oncol Clin N Am 30 (2021) xiii–xv
https://doi.org/10.1016/j.soc.2021.07.002
1055-3207/21/© 2021 Published by Elsevier Inc.

in pancreatic cancer are rooted in a broad integrated multidisciplinary approach with the surgeon as a central member of the treatment team.

I am grateful to have Dr Douglas Evans and Dr Susan Tsai as the guest editors of this issue of *Surgical Oncology Clinics of North America*. Dr Evans is the Chair of Surgery at the Medical College of Wisconsin where he holds the Donald C. Ausman Family Foundation Chair. Dr Evans has devoted his entire professional career to the research and treatment of pancreatic cancer. His interests include translational laboratory research in the biology of pancreatic cancer and in clinical trial development, having completed a number of investigator-initiated clinical trials. Dr Evans obtained his medical degree at Boston University and subsequently completed his residency at Dartmouth. He completed a Surgical Oncology Fellowship at The University of Texas MD Anderson Cancer Center. Dr Evans has served on various national medical advisory committees and has worked extensively with patient advocacy groups, including the Pancreatic Cancer Action Network and the Lustgarten Foundation. Dr Tsai is an Associate Professor in the Division of Surgical Oncology, Department of Surgery, and the Director of the LaBahn Pancreatic Cancer Program. She completed her medical school and residency training at the University of Michigan. During residency, she completed a Clinical Research Fellowship at the National Cancer Institute. After residency, she completed a Surgical Oncology Fellowship at the Johns Hopkins Hospital. Currently, Dr Tsai leads an active pancreatic cancer research program and serves as the Director of the Medical College of Wisconsin's Surgical Oncology Biorepository and Pancreatic Cancer Clinical Database. *Surgical Oncology Clinics of North America* could not have two more qualified individuals as co-guest editors of this issue on pancreatic cancer.

The issue covers a number of important topics, including pathology and molecular characteristics of pancreatic cancer, multimodality imaging, and advanced endoscopic techniques, all of which highlight the evolution in the treatment and surgical management of patients with pancreatic cancer. In addition, the issue also details current challenges and controversies related to neoadjuvant therapy as well as outlines new concepts related to systemic therapy as well as radiotherapy for pancreatic cancer. Furthermore, the authors do an outstanding job highlighting advances in precision medicine and the cutting-edge science currently underway to improve outcomes for patients with pancreatic cancer.

I owe Dr Evans and Dr Tsai much thanks for putting together such a fantastic team of oncology leaders to contribute to this issue of *Surgical Oncology Clinics of North America*. This group of authors has done a masterful job in highlighting the important and relevant aspects of caring for patients with pancreatic cancer. This issue of *Surgical Oncology Clinics of North America* will ensure that trainees and faculty are extremely knowledgeable in the latest information related to pancreatic cancer.

Again, I would like to thank Dr Evans and Dr Tsai as well as all the contributing authors for an outstanding issue of the *Surgical Oncology Clinics of North America*.

Timothy M. Pawlik, MD, MPH, MTS, PhD, FACS, FRACS (Hon.)
Department of Surgery
The Urban Meyer III and Shelley Meyer Chair for Cancer Research
Departments of Surgery, Oncology, and Health Services Management and Policy
The Ohio State University Wexner Medical Center
395 West 12th Avenue, Suite 670
Columbus, OH 43210, USA

E-mail address:
tim.pawlik@osumc.edu

REFERENCES

1. Khalaf N, El-Serag HB, Abrams HR. Burden of pancreatic cancer: from epidemiology to practice. Clin Gastroenterol Hepatol 2021;19(5):876–84.
2. Rhim AD, Mirek ET, Aiello NM, et al. EMT and dissemination precede pancreatic tumor formation. Cell 2012;148(1-2):349–61.
3. Conroy T, Desseigne F, Ycho M, et al. FOLFIRINOX versus gemcitabine for metastatic pancreatic cancer. N Engl J Med 2011;364:1817–25.

Preface

Updates on the Management of Pancreatic Cancer

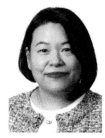 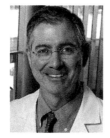

Susan Tsai, MD, MHS   Douglas B. Evans, MD
Editors

Management of pancreatic cancer has evolved rapidly over the past decade. The use of multimodality therapy has produced superior patient outcomes and has fueled the acceptance of neoadjuvant therapy as the standard approach to operable pancreatic cancer at most high-volume centers. The complexities of delivering neoadjuvant therapy requires the commitment of a multidisciplinary team. The focus of this issue is to highlight the importance of a multidisciplinary approach, and to that end, the issue is organized to provide a comprehensive overview of the management of pancreatic cancer from diagnosis to staging and treatment.

There have been significant scientific breakthroughs that have impacted the landscape of pancreatic cancer, and those advances will be highlighted in each article, from molecular profiling and tumor classification to robotic surgery. This issue of the *Surgical Oncology Clinics of North America* is broadly focused on the areas of diagnosis, treatment sequencing, and innovative surgical advances. Regarding diagnosis, the nuances of pancreatic cancer biology and subtype are discussed, the elements of state-of-the-art radiographic imaging and clinical staging are detailed, and the advances in endoscopic management of biliary obstruction and gastric outlet obstruction are reviewed. There remains considerable controversy in the optimal treatment sequencing of pancreatic cancer. The current practice and future landscape of systemic therapy, use of radiotherapy, promising novel therapeutics, and the adoption of precision medicine are reviewed as well. Finally, we conclude this issue with an update on both minimally invasive surgery for pancreatic cancer and vascular reconstruction at the time of pancreatectomy. Collectively, we hope this issue will serve as a useful reference for busy clinicians, clinical investigators, and scientists.

Surg Oncol Clin N Am 30 (2021) xvii–xviii
https://doi.org/10.1016/j.soc.2021.07.001
1055-3207/21/© 2021 Published by Elsevier Inc.

With great appreciation, we thank the authors for their generous contributions and expertise and the publishers for preparing this issue.

Susan Tsai, MD, MHS
LaBahn Pancreatic Cancer Program
Medical College of Wisconsin
8701 West Watertown Plank Road
Milwaukee, WI 53226-3596, USA

Douglas B. Evans, MD
Department of Surgery
Medical College of Wisconsin
8701 W Watertown Plank Road
Milwaukee, WI 53226-3596, USA

E-mail addresses:
stsai@mcw.edu (S. Tsai)
devans@mcw.edu (D.B. Evans)

Pathology and Molecular Characteristics of Pancreatic Cancer

Joseph F. Kearney, MD[a], Volkan Adsay, MD[b], Jen Jen Yeh, MD[c],*

KEYWORDS

- Pancreatic cancer • Tumor microenvironment • Pancreatic ductal adenocarcinoma

KEY POINTS

- Pancreatic ductal adenocarcinoma (PDAC) consists of both the tumor and the tumor microenvironment, both of which play an important role in patient outcomes.
- Understanding the genetic and transcriptomic drivers for each patient's tumor may help in tailoring therapies.
- The tumor and immune microenvironment of PDAC is complex and needs to be understood for therapy development.

INTRODUCTION

Most cancers of the pancreas are pancreatic ductal adenocarcinomas (PDAC). Thus, PDAC (and all its clinical characteristics, including its dismal prognosis) has become synonymous with "pancreas cancer."[1] However, it should be kept in mind that there is a whole host of other cancer types that occur in this organ. These cancers are classified by their cellular lineage: acinar cell carcinomas (acinar differentiation), neuroendocrine neoplasms (arising from the islets), solid-pseudopapillary neoplasms (showing no discernible cell lineage), and pancreatoblastomas (characterized by multiphenotypic differentiation including acinar endocrine and ductal). Mesenchymal neoplasms, such as gastrointestinal stromal tumors and lymphomas, can also occur in the pancreas. Cancers arising from the ampulla, duodenum, and bile ducts, as well as distant metastases to the pancreas from a remote organ, may present as tumors in the pancreas, but should be distinguished from primary PDACs. The ensuing text

[a] Surgery, University of North Carolina at Chapel Hill, 101 Manning Drive, 1150 Physicians Office Building, 21-245 Lineberger CB# 7213, Chapel Hill, NC 27599-7213, USA; [b] Department of Pathology, Koc University School of Medicine and KUTTAM Research Center, Koc University Hospital, Davutpasa Caddesi, Topkapi, Istanbul 34010, Turkey; [c] Surgery and Pharmacology, University of North Carolina at Chapel Hill, 101 Manning Drive, 1150 Physicians Office Building, 21-245 Lineberger CB# 7213, Chapel Hill, NC 27599-7213, USA
* Corresponding author.
E-mail address: jjyeh@med.unc.edu
Twitter: @yehlabUNC (J.J.Y.)

Surg Oncol Clin N Am 30 (2021) 609–619
https://doi.org/10.1016/j.soc.2021.06.003
surgonc.theclinics.com

focuses mostly on the "pancreas cancer," that is, PDAC, its precursors, and related carcinomas.

The cause of PDAC is unknown for most cases, but a small percentage (5%) of cases is attributed to genetic predisposition. Peutz-Jeghers patients (*STK11* gene alteration) have about a 75- to 135-fold increase; hereditary pancreatitis families (*PRSS1*) have about a roughly 50- to 60-fold increase; FAMM (*P16/CKN2A*) patients have about a 12- to 46-fold increase; Lynch patients have about a 7- to 8-fold increase, and other germline *BRCA*, *PALB2*, and *ATM* alterations have a less than 5-fold risk of developing PDAC,[2] leaving 95% of the cases unaccounted for. Some medical conditions, such as chronic pancreatitis, diabetes mellitus, peptic ulcer disease, periodontal disease, and prior cholecystectomy, have been found to have minimally increased risk (in the range of 2- to 5-fold)[3,4]; however, most patients have none of these diseases. Recently, anatomic variations of the pancreas and biliary ductal system have also been found to be associated with pancreas and biliary cancers, which may point to local chemical factors, especially bile, playing a potential role in pancreatic carcinogenesis.[5,6]

The understanding of molecular and genetic alterations involved in PDAC is rapidly expanding. Within the last decade, advancements in molecular biology and genetics coupled with advances in the fields of data science and machine learning have enabled researchers to provide meaningful insights into tumor biology. These advances in understanding are being augmented by the expanding armamentarium of available chemotherapy and biologics, which are on the cusp of bringing about an era of targeted therapies based on tumor biology.

Despite these advances, the 5-year survival of PDAC remains less than 10%. It has a dismal prognosis even when it is discovered in early stages, and it is projected to become the second leading cause of cancer deaths in the United States by 2030.[7] This review first discusses the histopathology of PDAC and other carcinomas of ductal lineage, followed by the molecular characteristics of the tumor microenvironment (TME) and their role in PDAC pathogenesis.

THE TUMOR
Histopathology

PDAC is characterized by invasive, widely separated small tubular (ductal) structures embedded in fibroinflammatory ("desmoplastic") stroma, which creates a scirrhous ill-defined lesion that is difficult to distinguish from chronic pancreatitis both radiologically and pathologically. The infiltration pattern is characteristically subtle, which often disallows it to form a well-defined mass, but rather a highly insidious infiltration that leads to peritoneal carcinomatosis with numerous small clusters, whereas the primary tumor may seemingly be relatively small. The richness of desmoplasia combined with the wide separation of carcinoma glands creates challenges for the genetic analysis of PDAC; this is because there often is very minimal carcinoma and abundant host tissue in a given tumor fragment. It should be noted that studies comparing "normal pancreas" with PDAC are not fair comparisons because the ducts, which are the normal counterparts of PDAC, are only a small component of normal pancreatic parenchyma; most of the pancreas tissue is composed of acini, which are a different cell type.

Other Carcinomas of Ductal Lineage

There are other pancreatic carcinomas of ductal origin that are related to PDAC, but also show substantial diversion from PDACs in many respects.[1,8] Determining how and why these carcinomas differ from PDAC may prove informative regarding the carcinogenesis of ordinary PDAC. *Morphologic variants* of PDAC, such as foamy gland, large duct, and vacuolated cell, likely represent some alteration in the cellular machinery of the PDAC cells, but the overall characteristics of these carcinomas do not substantially differ from that of PDACs.

The following carcinomas, which used to be classified as PDACs but are increasingly being viewed as different cancer types, appear to have different biologic and clinicopathologic characteristics. *Adenosquamous carcinomas* are thought to cluster with the "basallike" group in genomic profiling (which is also distinguished by low GATA6 and high CK5/6 and p40 expression) and are even more aggressive than ordinary PDACs, with rapid mortality. *Micropapillary carcinoma* is another aggressive ductal carcinoma that is characterized by reversal of cell polarity, with MUC1 decorating the stroma-facing surface of the cells instead of the luminal surface. *Colloid (mucinous noncystic) carcinomas* are less aggressive, with an incomparably better behavior with 5-year survival greater than 60%.[9] These carcinomas are very similar to colloid carcinomas of the breast and are characterized by diffuse expression of intestinal differentiation markers (CDX2/MUC2), which are not otherwise seen in PDACs nor other invasive carcinomas. The inhibitory effect of MUC2 gel-forming mucin combined with cells' confinement within the mucin pools is thought to account for their more favorable course. *Medullary carcinomas* are a very rare primary tumor of the pancreas[10] and often prove to be of ampullary origin. They are characterized by mismatch repair (MMR) deficiency, more indolent behavior, and an intense immune response that renders them candidates for immune checkpoint inhibitors.

Undifferentiated carcinomas are a heterogeneous group that are being characterized increasingly and are now recognized to have at least 3 distinct tumor types. *Rhabdoid* undifferentiated carcinomas[11] have been found to be driven by alterations in the SWItch/sucrose nonfermentable complex, characterized by loss of INI-1 and BRG, and there are various targeted therapies under investigation specifically for these aggressive tumors. *Osteoclastic giant cell carcinomas*[12] (sarcomatoid undifferentiated carcinomas with osteoclast) are a peculiar group that is characterized by osteoclast (CD68-positive bone resorption cells of macrophagic origin) infiltration to the tumor. Last, the *not otherwise specified* type of pleomorphic undifferentiated carcinomas expresses more epithelial mesenchymal transition markers than the osteoclastic types, and Snai2 has been found to have a central role in these sarcomatoid carcinomas.[13]

Tumoral Intraepithelial Neoplasms

Invasive cancers arising from tumoral intraepithelial neoplasms (adenoma-carcinoma sequence), namely, cystic and intraductal neoplasms (ie, intraductal papillary mucinous neoplasms, intraductal oncocytic papillary neoplasms, and intraductal tubulopapillary neoplasms) and mucinous cystic neoplasms, all have distinct clinicopathologic characteristics and molecular pathways.[14,15] Preliminary evidence suggests that even ordinary-type PDACs arising from these mass-forming preinvasive neoplasms appear to have distinct molecular and genetic characteristics and clinical behavior. There are also distinct pathways that exist in this generic group, such as the CDX2/MUC2-expressing intestinal pathway (colloid-type invasive carcinomas arising from intestinal type of intraductal papillary mucinous neoplasms). Intraductal oncocytic papillary neoplasm is also a distinct clinicopathologic entity[16] that was recently found to have a specific driver molecular alteration.[17] More studies are needed to further clarify this broad category of tumors.

DNA Mutations in Pancreatic Ductal Adenocarcinoma

KRAS is a small-molecule GTPase that is mutated in 94% of PDAC, resulting in persistent GTP-binding and constitutive activation of its downstream pathways that drive oncogenesis. Certain *KRAS* codon mutations may be associated with outcome.[18,19] Patients with wild-type *KRAS* tumors appear to have complementary mutations that activate either upstream or downstream KRAS effectors, illustrating the importance of this pathway.[20]

The key genetic mutations in the progression from PanIN to invasive PDAC are: *KRAS* (94%), *CDKN2A* (>90%), *TP53* (75%), and *SMAD4* (55%). The activating *KRAS* mutation is thought to be the earliest and can be found in PanINs.[21] After acquisition of a *KRAS* mutation, there is thought to be a selective pressure placed on the cells that induces and selects for the loss of the CDKN2A and TP53 tumor suppressors. SMAD4 is a downstream effector within the TGF-beta pathway. TGF-beta pathway activation results in both tumor-promoting and -suppressing roles that are carefully balanced. SMAD4 loss results in a shift in this balance toward tumor-promoting via KLF5 and SOX4 cooperation.[22]

BRCA1 and *BRCA2* are germline mutations that alter the DNA damage repair (DDR) pathway. Patients with *BRCA1/2* mutations benefit from treatment with platinum-based therapies.[23] In a recent study, poly(adenosine diphosphate-ribose) polymerase inhibition as maintenance therapy was shown to improve progression-free survival in patients with *BRCA1/2* mutations in the metastatic setting.[24] Analysis from the Know Your Tumor study showed that patients with somatic mutations in the DDR pathway also derive more benefit from platinum-based therapies.[23,25] MMR, characterized by mutations in *MLH1, MSH2, MSH6,* and *PMS2,* account for less than 1% of all PDACs.[26] In fact, a carcinoma that shows MMR loss in the head of the pancreas is much more likely to be of ampullary origin.[27] PDACs that show MMR deficiency may benefit from immunotherapy approaches.[28] As mentioned above, only 5% to 10% of patients with PDAC have a family history and other predisposing germline mutations (*ATM, CDKNA, CDKN2A, EPCAM, PALB2, PRSS1, STK11,* and *TP53*).[20]

Epigenetic Changes

DNA methylation

CpG islands refer to cytosine-guanine (C-G) dinucleotides where, over a length greater than 200 base-pairs, the GC content is greater than 50%. These regions in the genome are often found in mammalian promoters. C is prone to the acquisition of methyl groups via DNA methyltransferases. Methylation of the CpG islands in promoter regions results in suppression of gene transcription. *BNC1* and *ADAMTS1* are the most methylated genes in PDAC, and they are preferentially methylated in preneoplastic states. The evaluation of circulating free DNA for methylation patterns as biomarkers for PDAC is ongoing.[29]

Histone Modifications

Histones are the building blocks of the nucleosome, which provides a scaffolding for chromosomal DNA storage. Patterns of methylation and acetylation of lysine residues on histone tails are powerful regulators for gene expression, governing transcription and splicing. Recent work showed histone expression patterns for the *KLF4, SOX9,* and *ERBB2* transcription factors, whereas the hedgehog (Hh) pathway and tumor suppressor genes (*BRCA2* and *SMAD4*) were repressed.[30]

Noncoding RNAs

Newer areas of study in PDAC include noncoding (nc)RNAs, such as micro-RNA (miRNA) and long ncRNAs (lncRNA), in tumorigenesis. miRNA is small ncRNA that modulates translation of messenger RNAs. They are transcribed in the cell nucleus and undergo processing before associating with the RNA-induced silencing complex

(RISC). The miRNA then guides the RISC to the corresponding mRNA to suppress translation.[31] miRNAs can also be detected in the serum, and they are currently under investigation for use as biomarkers in PDAC.[32] lncRNAs are RNA transcripts greater than 200 base-pairs that are not translated into proteins. Their genes are primarily within the intergenic and intronic regions of the genome. The understanding of the role of lncRNAs in PDAC is in its infancy.

Transcriptomic Subtypes

Gene expression in PDAC has been studied with both tumor and TME gene expression patterns emerging. Currently, there are thought to be 2 tumor-intrinsic subtypes: basallike and classical.[33–37] Other subtype schemas (classical/quasimesenchymal/exocrine; squamous/progenitor/immunogenic/ADEX) overlap with the 2 tumor-intrinsic schema and may also define TME patterns.[34,36] The classical subtype is characterized by high GATA6 expression and extracellular mucin.[33] The basallike subtype is associated with decreased overall survival and a decreased response to FOLFIRINOX.[38] A predictive gene expression-based biomarker assay[39] is now being evaluated in clinical trials (NCT04683315), and GATA6 is being studied as an immunohistochemical marker.[40,41] Adenosquamous carcinomas of the pancreas are in the "basallike" subtype group.

THE TUMOR MICROENVIRONMENT

PDAC is uniquely characterized by a desmoplastic stroma that plays competing roles in promoting tumor growth and preventing tumor metastasis and invasion. A significant portion of research in the TME is dedicated to delineating how the stromal components promote these competing phenotypes and determining if targeting them can confer a more favorable outcome for patients. The TME consists of the extracellular matrix (ECM), cancer-associated fibroblasts (CAFs), tumor microvasculature, neurons, and adaptive and innate immune cells. The bidirectional interaction of tumor cells with the TME is highly complex, with both protumorigenic and tumor-inhibiting properties.

The Extracellular Matrix

Key proteins contributing to the ECM in PDAC are collagen (type I, II, and IV), hyaluronic acid, and fibronectin. The dense ECM contributes to a high intratumoral oncotic pressure, which in turn collapses smaller blood vessels and inhibits drug diffusion from the circulation into the tumor.[42] In a trial of PEGPH20 (PEGylated Recombinant Human Hyaluronidase) with mFOLFIRINOX, many patients had adverse reactions to PEGPH20, and those who tolerated therapy did not show improvement in tumor response or overall survival.[43] The HALO trials evaluated PEGPH with gemcitabine and nab-paclitaxel,[44,45] but despite early promising data, it failed to meet its primary endpoint in phase 3 trials.[46] Despite early failures in ECM-directed regimens, there are promising results from in vitro and mouse studies targeting collagen metabolism[47] and ECM synthesis.[48]

Neural Tissue

Perineural invasion is a common pathologic finding and a risk factor for recurrence after surgery, and tumors have a high density of neurons in them.[49] With careful inspection and adequate sampling, many PDACs prove to have neural invasion. Axonogenesis is triggered by the release of tumor-derived netrins and promote neural outgrowth into the tumor, and this, in turn, promotes an inflammatory response within the tumor, in tumor growth, and in invasion.[50,51] Understanding the neurobiology in PDAC (and other solid tumors) may provide opportunities for intervention.

Vasculature

Many PDAC specimens exhibit vascular invasion of the small-caliber vessels. When PDACs infiltrate vasculature, tumor cells start to line the endothelial surface and ultimately form ductlike structures that can be indistinguishable from PanINs in histologic sections. This peculiar ability is unique to PDAC. High intratumoral pressure reduces tumor perfusion, resulting in a hypoxic environment.[52] Tumor hypoxia results in a disorganized, pericyte-poor neovascularization by vasculogenesis driven by vascular endothelial growth factor A (VEGF-A) and recruitment of endothelial progenitor cells.[53] Increasing tumor pericyte coverage improves vessel integrity,[54] and VEGF inhibition enables an adaptive immune cell response to the tumor from improved adhesion and transmigration[55] and improves drug delivery. Phase 3 trials using antiangiogenic therapies have failed to meet primary endpoints for overall survival[52]; however, there is cautious optimism for the role of pairing these agents with immune-checkpoint blockade.[42]

Cancer-Associated Fibroblasts

CAFs arise predominantly from pancreatic stellate cells, as well as from bone marrow–derived mesenchymal stem cells, and their formation has been shown to be secondary to tumor signals.[56–59] CAFs that differentially express αSMA (myCAFs) have contractile properties and are thought to restrain PDAC tumor growth. CAFs that differentially express PDGFR-alpha and secrete chemokines and interleukins (IL-1 and IL-6) are termed inflammatory CAFs (iCAFs).[56,60] There are also antigen-presenting CAFs (apCAFs) that play a role in immune modulation by exhibiting major histocompatibility complex–II and binding with CD4+ T cells.[61] CAFs may regulate PDAC phenotype and tumor cell survival through a variety of mechanisms. They provide nutritional support to tumor cells,[62] modulate the immune environment within the TME,[61,63] and secrete several growth factors that promote neovascularization and tumor growth.[63] Furthermore, an increasing number of studies show that CAFs may alter response to therapy.[64–67]

CAF-directed therapies have been unsuccessful to date. An early attempt to modulate tumor-stroma crosstalk in PDAC through Hh inhibition had to be terminated prematurely because patients treated with an Hh inhibitor had unexpectedly poor outcomes compared with gemcitabine alone.[68]

The Immune System

The immune system is an active area of investigation in PDAC. Infiltration of lymphoid cells into PDAC tumors is associated with improved survival.[69] This beneficial cytotoxic effect of T cells may be blunted by subsequent qualitative dysfunction, which is mediated by regulatory T cells, myeloid-derived suppressor cells (MDSCs), tumor-associated macrophages (TAMs), and inhibitory cytokines.[70] These dysfunctional intratumoral T cells also upregulate checkpoint inhibitory receptors, such as the programmed cell death receptor 1 (PD-1).[68] Cells of myeloid lineage, such as TAMs and MDSCs, enable immune evasion in PDAC. TAMs exhibit M1 (proinflammatory) and M2 (anti-inflammatory) polarization states and mediate therapy resistance. MDSCs are implicated in shifting TAM polarization to the M2 phenotype and T cells to a T-regulatory phenotype. They are also responsible for PD-1–PD-L1 checkpoint activation.[68] To date, single-agent checkpoint inhibitors have not been shown to be effective treatment in PDAC with several studies suggesting that a multipronged approach will be needed.[71]

SUMMARY

PDAC comprises an interplay of numerous cell types the role of which in the overall tumor behavior cannot be fully understood in isolation. Although most cases of PDAC arise from a series of genetic mutations, the epigenetic modifications play a major role in the overall tumor behavior. The importance of the TME is increasingly recognized. Although therapies targeting the TME have been disappointing, evolving understanding of this complex biology provides hope for more therapeutic options. Rare cancer types that are related to but also different from PDAC, such as colloid, medullary, osteoclastic, and rhabdoid, are proving to also have distinct genetic molecular characteristics. Understanding the mechanism of these tumors may shed light on the carcinogenesis of the more conventional PDAC. Recent studies illustrating that anatomic variations and even bile may have a major role in pancreatobiliary cancer formation have opened a new platform for researchers to focus on. As PDAC ascends the list of cancer-related mortality in the United States, it is imperative that we continue to develop and improve therapeutic options by investigating these various possibilities.

CLINICS CARE POINTS

- Germline mutations that increase risk for pancreatic ductal adenocarcinoma are *STK11, PRSS1, P16/CKN2A, BRCA, PALB2, ATM, MSH1, MSH2, MLHL, EPCAM,* and *PMS2.*
- Adenosquamous, colloid, and medullary carcinomas are increasingly being viewed as different cancer types, with different biologic and clinicopathologic characteristics.
- Patients with germline mutations in BRCA may benefit from both poly(adenosine diphosphate-ribose) polymerase inhibition and platinum-based therapy as maintenance chemotherapy, and patients with somatic mutations in the DNA damage repair pathways benefit from platinum-based therapies.
- Patients with mismatch repair mutations may benefit from immunotherapies.
- There are 2 tumor-intrinsic subtypes in pancreatic ductal adenocarcinoma: basallike and classical. The basallike subtype confers a worse prognosis and diminished response to FOLFIRINOX.
- The extracellular matrix provides a nutritional source to pancreatic ductal adenocarcinoma tumors and may inhibit drug delivery.
- Known cancer-associated fibroblast subpopulations are myCAFs, iCAFs, and apCAFs. The iCAFs and apCAFs appear to work together to promote tumor growth and immune evasion, whereas the myCAFs may restrain tumor growth.
- Myeloid cells create a dysfunctional immune response within the tumor.

DISCLOSURE

JJY is an inventor of PurIST which has been licensed to GeneCentric Technologies.

FUNDING

This study was funded by R01-CA199062 (JJY) and T32-CA244125 (JFK).

REFERENCES

1. Mostafa ME, Erbarut-Seven I, Pehlivanoglu B, et al. Pathologic classification of "pancreatic cancers": current concepts and challenges. Chin Clin Oncol 2017; 6(6):59.

2. Pitot HC, Riegel IL. The McArdle Laboratory for Cancer Research. Bioessays 1987;6(3):138–40.

3. Maisonneuve P, Lowenfels AB. Risk factors for pancreatic cancer: a summary review of meta-analytical studies. Int J Epidemiol 2015;44(1):186–98.

4. Maisonneuve P, Amar S, Lowenfels AB. Periodontal disease, edentulism, and pancreatic cancer: a meta-analysis. Ann Oncol 2017;28(5):985–95.

5. Midhagen G, Järnerot G, Kraaz W. Adult coeliac disease within a defined geographic area in Sweden. A study of prevalence and associated diseases. Scand J Gastroenterol 1988;23(8):1000–4.

6. Muraki T, Reid MD, Pehlivanoglu B, et al. Variant anatomy of the biliary system as a cause of pancreatic and peri-ampullary cancers. HPB (Oxford) 2020;22(12):1675–85.

7. Rahib L, Smith BD, Aizenberg R, et al. Projecting cancer incidence and deaths to 2030: the unexpected burden of thyroid, liver, and pancreas cancers in the United States. Cancer Res 2014;74(11):2913–21.

8. Bazzichetto C, Luchini C, Conciatori F, et al. Morphologic and molecular landscape of pancreatic cancer variants as the basis of new therapeutic strategies for precision oncology. Int J Mol Sci 2020;21(22).

9. Adsay NV, Pierson C, Sarkar F, et al. Colloid (mucinous noncystic) carcinoma of the pancreas. Am J Surg Pathol 2001;25(1):26–42.

10. Wilentz RE, Goggins M, Redston M, et al. Genetic, immunohistochemical, and clinical features of medullary carcinoma of the pancreas: a newly described and characterized entity. Am J Pathol 2000;156(5):1641–51.

11. Agaimy A, Haller F, Frohnauer J, et al. Pancreatic undifferentiated rhabdoid carcinoma: KRAS alterations and SMARCB1 expression status define two subtypes. Mod Pathol 2015;28(2):248–60.

12. Muraki T, Reid MD, Basturk O, et al. Undifferentiated carcinoma with osteoclastic giant cells of the pancreas: clinicopathologic analysis of 38 cases highlights a more protracted clinical course than currently appreciated. Am J Surg Pathol 2016;40(9):1203–16.

13. Mattiolo P, Fiadone G, Paolino G, et al. Epithelial-mesenchymal transition in undifferentiated carcinoma of the pancreas with and without osteoclast-like giant cells. Virchows Arch 2021;478(2):319–26.

14. Noë M, Niknafs N, Fischer CG, et al. Genomic characterization of malignant progression in neoplastic pancreatic cysts. Nat Commun 2020;11(1):4085.

15. Adsay V, Mino-Kenudson M, Furukawa T, et al. Pathologic evaluation and reporting of intraductal papillary mucinous neoplasms of the pancreas and other tumoral intraepithelial neoplasms of pancreatobiliary tract: recommendations of Verona consensus meeting. Ann Surg 2016;263(1):162–77.

16. Basturk O, Khayyata S, Klimstra DS, et al. Preferential expression of MUC6 in oncocytic and pancreatobiliary types of intraductal papillary neoplasms highlights a pyloropancreatic pathway, distinct from the intestinal pathway, in pancreatic carcinogenesis. Am J Surg Pathol 2010;34(3):364–70.

17. Vyas M, Hechtman JF, Zhang Y, et al. DNAJB1-PRKACA fusions occur in oncocytic pancreatic and biliary neoplasms and are not specific for fibrolamellar hepatocellular carcinoma. Mod Pathol 2020;33(4):648–56.

18. Bournet B, Muscari F, Buscail C, et al. KRAS G12D mutation subtype is a prognostic factor for advanced pancreatic adenocarcinoma. Clin Transl Gastroenterol 2016;7:e157.

19. Witkiewicz AK, McMillan EA, Balaji U, et al. Whole-exome sequencing of pancreatic cancer defines genetic diversity and therapeutic targets. Nat Commun 2015; 6:6744.

20. andrew_aguirre@dfci.harvard.edu CGARNEa, Network CGAR. Integrated genomic characterization of pancreatic ductal adenocarcinoma. Cancer Cell 2017;32(2):185–203.e113.

21. Iacobuzio-Donahue CA, Velculescu VE, Wolfgang CL, et al. Genetic basis of pancreas cancer development and progression: insights from whole-exome and whole-genome sequencing. Clin Cancer Res 2012;18(16):4257–65.

22. Shen W, Tao GQ, Zhang Y, et al. TGF-β in pancreatic cancer initiation and progression: two sides of the same coin. Cell Biosci 2017;7:39.

23. Pishvaian MJ, Blais EM, Brody JR, et al. Outcomes in patients with pancreatic adenocarcinoma with genetic mutations in DNA damage response pathways: results from the Know Your Tumor program. JCO Precision Oncol 2019;(3):1–10.

24. Golan T, Hammel P, Reni M, et al. Maintenance olaparib for germline. N Engl J Med 2019;381(4):317–27.

25. Pishvaian MJ, Blais EM, Brody JR, et al. Overall survival in patients with pancreatic cancer receiving matched therapies following molecular profiling: a retrospective analysis of the Know Your Tumor registry trial. Lancet Oncol 2020; 21(4):508–18.

26. Luchini C, Brosens LAA, Wood LD, et al. Comprehensive characterisation of pancreatic ductal adenocarcinoma with microsatellite instability: histology, molecular pathology and clinical implications. Gut 2021;70(1):148–56.

27. Xue Y, Balci S, Aydin Mericoz C, et al. Frequency and clinicopathologic associations of DNA mismatch repair protein deficiency in ampullary carcinoma: routine testing is indicated. Cancer 2020;126(21):4788–99.

28. Grant RC, Denroche R, Jang GH, et al. Clinical and genomic characterisation of mismatch repair deficient pancreatic adenocarcinoma. Gut Published Online First: 15 September 2020. https://doi.org/10.1136/gutjnl-2020-320730.

29. Brancaccio M, Natale F, Falco G, et al. Cell-free DNA methylation: the new frontiers of pancreatic cancer biomarkers' discovery. Genes (Basel) 2019;11(1).

30. Lomberk G, Blum Y, Nicolle R, et al. Distinct epigenetic landscapes underlie the pathobiology of pancreatic cancer subtypes. Nat Commun 2018;9(1):1978.

31. Daoud AZ, Mulholland EJ, Cole G, et al. MicroRNAs in pancreatic cancer: biomarkers, prognostic, and therapeutic modulators. BMC Cancer 2019;19(1):1130.

32. Abue M, Yokoyama M, Shibuya R, et al. Circulating miR-483-3p and miR-21 is highly expressed in plasma of pancreatic cancer. Int J Oncol 2015;46(2):539–47.

33. Moffitt RA, Marayati R, Flate EL, et al. Virtual microdissection identifies distinct tumor- and stroma-specific subtypes of pancreatic ductal adenocarcinoma. Nat Genet 2015;47(10):1168–78.

34. Collisson EA, Bailey P, Chang DK, et al. Molecular subtypes of pancreatic cancer. Nat Rev Gastroenterol Hepatol 2019;16(4):207–20.

35. Maurer C, Holmstrom SR, He J, et al. Experimental microdissection enables functional harmonisation of pancreatic cancer subtypes. Gut 2019;68(6):1034–43.

36. Bailey P, Chang DK, Nones K, et al. Genomic analyses identify molecular subtypes of pancreatic cancer. Nature 2016;531(7592):47–52.

37. Puleo F, Nicolle R, Blum Y, et al. Stratification of pancreatic ductal adenocarcinomas based on tumor and microenvironment features. Gastroenterology 2018; 155(6):1999–2013.e3.

38. Aung KL, Fischer SE, Denroche RE, et al. Genomics-driven precision medicine for advanced pancreatic cancer: early results from the COMPASS Trial. Clin Cancer Res 2018;24(6):1344–54.

39. Rashid NU, Peng XL, Jin C, et al. Purity independent subtyping of tumors (PurIST), a clinically robust, single-sample classifier for tumor subtyping in pancreatic cancer. Clin Cancer Res 2020;26(1):82–92.

40. O'Kane GM, Grunwald BT, Jang GH, et al. GATA6 expression distinguishes classical and basal-like subtypes in advanced pancreatic cancer. Clin Cancer Res 2020;26(18):4901–10.

41. Brunton H, Caligiuri G, Cunningham R, et al. HNF4A and GATA6 loss reveals therapeutically actionable subtypes in pancreatic cancer. Cell Rep 2020;31(6): 107625.

42. Hosein AN, Brekken RA, Maitra A. Pancreatic cancer stroma: an update on therapeutic targeting strategies. Nat Rev Gastroenterol Hepatol 2020;17(8):487–505.

43. Ramanathan RK, McDonough SL, Philip PA, et al. Phase IB/II randomized study of FOLFIRINOX plus pegylated recombinant human hyaluronidase versus FOLFIRINOX alone in patients with metastatic pancreatic adenocarcinoma: SWOG S1313. J Clin Oncol 2019;37(13):1062–9.

44. Hingorani SR, Zheng L, Bullock AJ, et al. HALO 202: randomized phase II study of PEGPH20 plus Nab-Paclitaxel/Gemcitabine versus Nab-Paclitaxel/Gemcitabine in patients with untreated, metastatic pancreatic ductal adenocarcinoma. J Clin Oncol 2018;36(4):359–66.

45. Doherty GJ, Tempero M, Corrie PG. HALO-109-301: a phase III trial of PEGPH20 (with gemcitabine and nab-paclitaxel) in hyaluronic acid-high stage IV pancreatic cancer. Future Oncol 2018;14(1):13–22.

46. Hakim N, Patel R, Devoe C, et al. Why HALO 301 failed and implications for treatment of pancreatic cancer. Pancreas (Fairfax) 2019;3(1):e1–4.

47. Olivares O, Mayers JR, Gouirand V, et al. Collagen-derived proline promotes pancreatic ductal adenocarcinoma cell survival under nutrient limited conditions. Nat Commun 2017;8:16031.

48. Vennin C, Chin VT, Warren SC, et al. Transient tissue priming via ROCK inhibition uncouples pancreatic cancer progression, sensitivity to chemotherapy, and metastasis. Sci Transl Med 2017;9(384).

49. Demir IE, Friess H, Ceyhan GO. Neural plasticity in pancreatitis and pancreatic cancer. Nat Rev Gastroenterol Hepatol 2015;12(11):649–59.

50. Wang W, Li L, Chen N, et al. Nerves in the tumor microenvironment: origin and effects. Front Cell Dev Biol 2020;8:601738.

51. Stopczynski RE, Normolle DP, Hartman DJ, et al. Neuroplastic changes occur early in the development of pancreatic ductal adenocarcinoma. Cancer Res 2014;74(6):1718–27.

52. Li S, Xu HX, Wu CT, et al. Angiogenesis in pancreatic cancer: current research status and clinical implications. Angiogenesis 2019;22(1):15–36.

53. Vizio B, Novarino A, Giacobino A, et al. Pilot study to relate clinical outcome in pancreatic carcinoma and angiogenic plasma factors/circulating mature/progenitor endothelial cells: preliminary results. Cancer Sci 2010;101(11):2448–54.

54. McCarty MF, Somcio RJ, Stoeltzing O, et al. Overexpression of PDGF-BB decreases colorectal and pancreatic cancer growth by increasing tumor pericyte content. J Clin Invest 2007;117(8):2114–22.

55. Shrimali RK, Yu Z, Theoret MR, et al. Antiangiogenic agents can increase lymphocyte infiltration into tumor and enhance the effectiveness of adoptive immunotherapy of cancer. Cancer Res 2010;70(15):6171–80.

56. Öhlund D, Handly-Santana A, Biffi G, et al. Distinct populations of inflammatory fibroblasts and myofibroblasts in pancreatic cancer. J Exp Med 2017;214(3): 579–96.
57. Kabashima-Niibe A, Higuchi H, Takaishi H, et al. Mesenchymal stem cells regulate epithelial-mesenchymal transition and tumor progression of pancreatic cancer cells. Cancer Sci 2013;104(2):157–64.
58. Bhagat TD, Von Ahrens D, Dawlaty M, et al. Lactate-mediated epigenetic reprogramming regulates formation of human pancreatic cancer-associated fibroblasts. Elife 2019;8.
59. Somerville TD, Biffi G, Daßler-Plenker J, et al. Squamous trans-differentiation of pancreatic cancer cells promotes stromal inflammation. Elife 2020;9.
60. Pereira BA, Vennin C, Papanicolaou M, et al. CAF subpopulations: a new reservoir of stromal targets in pancreatic cancer. Trends Cancer 2019;5(11):724–41.
61. Elyada E, Bolisetty M, Laise P, et al. Cross-species single-cell analysis of pancreatic ductal adenocarcinoma reveals antigen-presenting cancer-associated fibroblasts. Cancer Discov 2019;9(8):1102–23.
62. Sousa CM, Biancur DE, Wang X, et al. Pancreatic stellate cells support tumour metabolism through autophagic alanine secretion. Nature 2016;536(7617): 479–83.
63. Sahai E, Astsaturov I, Cukierman E, et al. A framework for advancing our understanding of cancer-associated fibroblasts. Nat Rev Cancer 2020;20(3):174–86.
64. McMillin DW, Delmore J, Weisberg E, et al. Tumor cell-specific bioluminescence platform to identify stroma-induced changes to anticancer drug activity. Nat Med 2010;16(4):483–9.
65. Olive KP, Jacobetz MA, Davidson CJ, et al. Inhibition of Hedgehog signaling enhances delivery of chemotherapy in a mouse model of pancreatic cancer. Science 2009;324(5933):1457–61.
66. Sherman MH, Yu RT, Engle DD, et al. Vitamin D receptor-mediated stromal reprogramming suppresses pancreatitis and enhances pancreatic cancer therapy. Cell 2014;159(1):80–93.
67. Toste PA, Nguyen AH, Kadera BE, et al. Chemotherapy-induced inflammatory gene signature and protumorigenic phenotype in pancreatic CAFs via stress-associated MAPK. Mol Cancer Res 2016;14(5):437–47.
68. Neesse A, Bauer CA, Ohlund D, et al. Stromal biology and therapy in pancreatic cancer: ready for clinical translation? Gut 2019;68(1):159–71.
69. Fukunaga A, Miyamoto M, Cho Y, et al. CD8+ tumor-infiltrating lymphocytes together with CD4+ tumor-infiltrating lymphocytes and dendritic cells improve the prognosis of patients with pancreatic adenocarcinoma. Pancreas 2004; 28(1):e26–31.
70. Bailey P, Chang DK, Forget MA, et al. Exploiting the neoantigen landscape for immunotherapy of pancreatic ductal adenocarcinoma. Sci Rep 2016;6:35848.
71. Henriksen A, Dyhl-Polk A, Chen I, et al. Checkpoint inhibitors in pancreatic cancer. Cancer Treat Rev 2019;78:17–30.

Multimodality Imaging for the Staging of Pancreatic Cancer

Martin McKinney, MD[a], Michael O. Griffin, MD, PhD[a,b],
Parag P. Tolat, MD[a,b],*

KEYWORDS

- Pancreatic cancer • Staging • Computed tomography
- Magnetic resonance imaging • Neoadjuvant therapy • Indeterminate liver lesions
- Structured reporting

KEY POINTS

- A pancreatic protocol, dual-phase, contrast-enhanced, multidetector computed tomography examination is the cornerstone of initial staging of pancreatic ductal adenocarcinoma.
- Several imaging techniques can be important for staging pancreatic ductal adenocarcinoma and supplement the pancreatic protocol computed tomography scans.
- The accuracy of imaging in assessing response to neoadjuvant therapy is limited.
- Structured reporting of the staging computed tomography scan leads to more complete and accurate staging of pancreatic ductal adenocarcinoma compared with a free-form radiology dictation.

INTRODUCTION

Imaging plays a key role in the diagnosis, staging, and follow-up of pancreatic ductal adenocarcinoma (PDAC), with the pancreatic protocol dual-phase multidetector computed tomography (CT) scan being the imaging examination of choice. A CT scan is highly accurate for pancreatic tumor detection, assessment of resectability, and detection of metastatic disease. This article reviews key principles of the acquisition, interpretation, and reporting of PDAC imaging with CT scanning, as well as highlights potential roles for newer and supplemental imaging technologies such as dual-energy CT scanning, MRI, and PET, including PET/CT scanning and

[a] Department of Radiology, Medical College of Wisconsin, 9200 West Wisconsin Avenue, Milwaukee, WI 53226, USA; [b] Department of and Surgery, Medical College of Wisconsin, 9200 West Wisconsin Avenue, Milwaukee, WI 53226, USA
* Corresponding author. Department of Radiology, Medical College of Wisconsin, 9200 West Wisconsin Avenue, Milwaukee, WI 53226.
E-mail address: ptolat@mcw.edu

Surg Oncol Clin N Am 30 (2021) 621–637
https://doi.org/10.1016/j.soc.2021.06.006
1055-3207/21/© 2021 Elsevier Inc. All rights reserved.
surgonc.theclinics.com

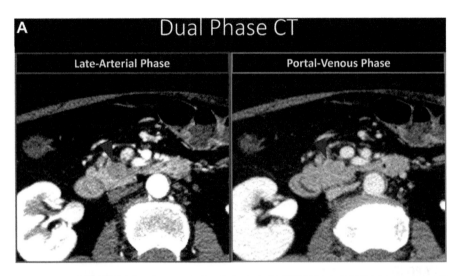

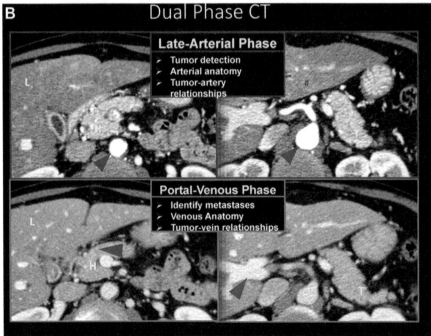

Fig. 1. (A) Late arterial and portal venous phases at the level of the pancreatic head. There is a subtle resectable low-attenuating mass (adenocarcinoma) confined entirely to the pancreas (*purple arrowhead*) seen only in the late arterial phase contrasted against the enhancing normal pancreatic parenchyma. The mass is completely invisible on the portal venous phase. (B) Late arterial and portal venous phases of the pancreas from head (H) to tail (T). In the late arterial phase, there is avid enhancement of the aorta (*red arrowhead*) and visceral arteries (#), and diffuse pancreatic parenchymal enhancement. In the portal venous phase, there is homogenous enhancement of the portal vein (*blue arrowhead*) and liver (L).

PET/MRI. In addition, we discuss the importance of structured interpretation and reporting of imaging examinations for providing the most complete and accurate assessment of tumor stage and resectability.

TECHNIQUE
Multidetector Computed Tomography Scan

A multidetector CT scan with a "dual-phase" pancreas protocol is the cornerstone of initial staging of newly diagnosed PDAC. The pancreas protocol is performed with intravenous (IV) contrast and acquired in both the pancreatic (or late arterial) and hepatic (or portal venous) phases, giving the name "dual phase." Accurate acquisition timing of the 2 scans after IV contrast administration is paramount to optimizing the conspicuity of the pancreatic tumor and for the detection of extrapancreatic metastatic disease. The patient also drinks a neutral contrast agent immediately before the scan to distend the duodenum and improve delineation of normal anatomy and any potential periampullary tumors. The neutral contrast agent typically is simple drinking water, but a 0.1% (w/v) barium sulfate suspension such as NeuLumEX (formerly VoLumen) (Bracco Diagnostics) or a sorbitol/mannitol mixture such as Breeza (Beekley Medical) can also be used. It is critical that the typical iodinated positive contrast agents used for most CT examinations not be used, because these agents can obscure the anatomy in the region of the pancreatic head and ampulla in addition to limiting the value of additional postprocessing techniques.[1–4]

Peak enhancement of the pancreas occurs during the late arterial phase, the key phase for pancreatic tumor detection. This phase provides the greatest conspicuity of an adenocarcinoma owing to the contrast between the avidly enhancing normal pancreatic parenchyma and the relatively hypoenhancing tumor (**Fig. 1**A). The late arterial phase is also the best phase for analyzing the peripancreatic arterial anatomy and its relationship to the tumor (**Fig. 1**B). The late arterial phase occurs approximately 25 to 35 seconds after the IV contrast bolus is delivered to the patient. The scan is completed through the entire abdomen during a single breath hold. The acquired late arterial phase images are then used to detect and measure the primary pancreatic tumor, assess visceral arterial anatomy and anomalies, and assess tumor–arterial involvement.[1–4]

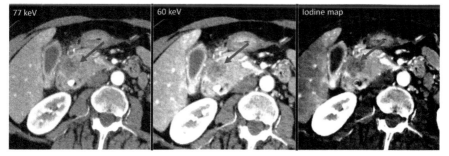

Fig. 2. Dual-energy CT scan improves lesion detection. Given atomic characteristics, iodine become brighter (or hyperenhancing) on lower energy reconstructed images. The pancreatic mass (*red arrow*) is more easily seen as the image reconstructions are adjusted (lower keV and iodine map images) to maximize enhancement of iodine in comparison to a hypoenhancing adenocarcinoma, providing better contrast between the tumor and adjacent normal pancreas.

Both manual and automated methods can be used for timing the late arterial phase acquisition. The simplest method is to use a fixed scan delay of 25 to 30 seconds after administration of the contrast bolus; however, more robust methods are available (ie, bolus tracking/triggering vs minitest bolus). Automated bolus tracking techniques monitor for contrast arrival in the aorta and then start the scan after a short delay. The timing bolus technique determines the time to arrival in the aorta of a small contrast test bolus, and this time is used to prescribe the scan delay for the full contrast injection. Both the bolus tracking and test bolus techniques provide an individualized approach tailored to each patient's cardiac output and are superior to a fixed scan delay.[3,5,6]

The second phase, or portal venous phase, is acquired with a delay of 60 to 70 seconds after the IV contrast bolus. Most providers are accustomed to seeing the portal venous phase on a CT scan because it is used for the majority of routine abdomen and pelvis imaging that only requires a single phase of contrast. This phase is the most

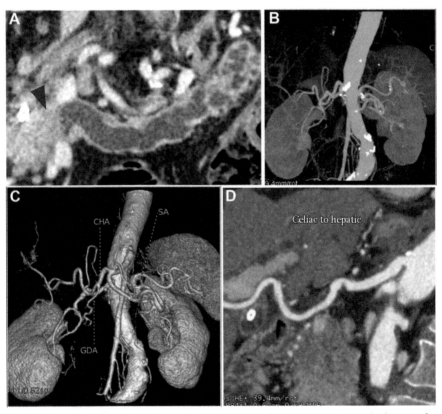

Fig. 3. Three-dimensional (3D) reconstructed images demonstrating curved planar reformats of the pancreatic and vascular anatomy: long axis view of the pancreatic duct (*A*). Vascular anatomy highlighted with maximum intensity projection image (*B*), 3D volume rendered image (*C*), and curved planar CTA image following the celiac to hepatic artery (*D*). Note the mass in the pancreatic head (*purple arrowhead* in [*A*] obstructing the duct). Normal (type 1) arterial anatomy is depicted maximum intensity projection (*B*) and 3D volume-rendered (*C*) images. No evident tumor abutment of the celiac and hepatic arteries on the arterial curved plane image (*D*).

helpful for assessing venous anatomy and anomalies, patency of the venous structures, and tumor–venous involvement (see **Fig. 1**B). This phase is also the best phase for detecting metastatic disease to the liver, lymph nodes, and peritoneum. The field of view during the second phase includes the lung bases through the pelvis and provides a general survey of the abdomen and pelvis.[1–4]

Dual energy CT (DECT) scanning is a newer technology that is being increasingly used for various applications throughout radiology.[7,8] The essence of a dual energy CT scan lies in the acquisition of images using 2 different photon energies during the same scan (eg, 80 and 120 kVp). DECT scans can provide additional information on tissue composition as well as improve the conspicuity of iodine-containing substances. In the pancreas, a DECT scan increases the contrast between normal parenchyma and tumor compared with a single energy CT scan, thereby increasing tumor conspicuity (**Fig. 2**). A DECT scan is generally used during the late arterial phase to improve pancreatic tumor detection; however, DECT scanning may also improve detection of liver metastases when used in the portal venous phase.[3,9]

In addition to improving pancreatic tumor detection, DECT scanning can decrease metal artifacts and is particularly useful in patients with metallic biliary stents, surgical clips, or embolic coils in the areas of interest. In addition, virtual noncontrast images can be reconstructed from the contrast-enhanced data without the need for a dedicated unenhanced image acquisition. A DECT scan can also improve the overall contrast in an image if the contrast bolus was suboptimal, through the use of reconstructed low kV virtual monoenergetic images. DECT scans can even allow for a lower IV contrast volume to be administered, which is particularly helpful for patients with decreased renal function.[3,7–9]

Three-dimensional (3D) reformations can be particularly helpful for assessing pancreatic tumors and the peripancreatic vascular anatomy. At the authors' institution, subvolume maximum intensity projections, 3D volume-rendered reformations, and curved–planar reformations are created by dedicated 3D technologists (**Fig. 3**). Subvolume maximum intensity projections of the late arterial and portal venous phases and 3D volume-rendered images of the arteries provide an overview of the

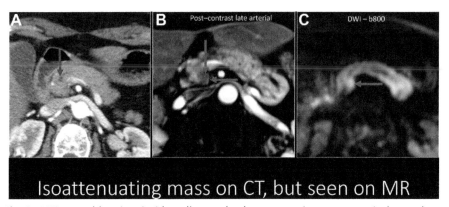

Fig. 4. A 73-year-old patient incidentally noted to have a prominent pancreatic duct on lumbar spine MRI. A focal prominent pancreatic duct (*red arrow*) was noted on a follow-up CT scan (*A*) without an associated measurable obstructing lesion. The patient went on to abdominal MR with postcontrast (*B*) and diffusion weighted images (*C*) demonstrating a subtle, small, hypoenhancing, diffusion restricting, obstructing mass (*purple arrows*). The patient went on to endoscopic ultrasound examination/FNA with final pathology of adenocarcinoma.

arterial and venous vasculature and highlight anatomic variants. Curved–planar reformations of the celiac, hepatic, and superior mesenteric arteries can highlight any tumor contact of the arteries, and curved–planar reformations of the pancreatic duct can highlight small tumors causing ductal obstruction.[1–4,10]

MRI

A contrast-enhanced, pancreas protocol CT scan is the preferred modality for the staging and follow-up of pancreatic cancer owing to its high spatial resolution and good tissue contrast. Although MRI offers improved tissue contrast compared with a CT scan, it suffers from lower spatial resolution and motion artifacts that can impair the assessment of tumor–vascular relationships. However, MRI has an important role in certain situations. In patients unable to receive iodinated contrast material for a CT scan owing to allergy or poor renal function, a contrast-enhanced MRI with magnetic resonance cholangiopancreatography (MRCP) is the modality of choice for tumor staging and follow-up. In those patients without a contraindication to a contrast-enhanced CT scan, MRI is best used as a problem-solving tool. The inherently high soft tissue contrast of an MRI can provide better detection of lesions that are not seen well with a CT scan, including small tumors or tumors that enhance similar to normal pancreas on a CT scan (ie, the small proportion of adenocarcinomas that are isoattenuating rather than hypoattenuating relative to normal pancreas) **(Fig. 4)**. In patients with a high clinical suspicion for pancreatic cancer but without an evident lesion on CT scan, MRI can be a useful adjunct with improved sensitivity of tumor detection. In addition, MRI can allow further evaluation of liver lesions detected on a CT scan, including those lesions with nonspecific imaging features on a CT scan or those lesions that are too small to characterize on a CT scan. MRI/MRCP also provides improved visualization and assessment of the intrahepatic and extrahepatic biliary ductal system and pancreatic duct compared with a CT scan.[1,3,9,11]

Briefly, MRI sequences to evaluate pancreatic cancer include T2-weighted fast-spin echo with and without fat saturation, T1-weighted in-phase and opposed-phase gradient echo, T1-weighted gradient echo with fat suppression without and with dynamic postcontrast imaging, diffusion-weighted imaging (DWI) with apparent diffusion coefficient map, and 3D MRCP, all acquired through the upper abdomen.[1,3] All of these acquisitions require breath-holding or respiratory gating, which can be

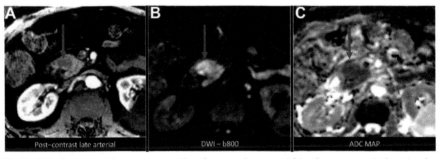

Fig. 5. MRI demonstrating a pancreatic adenocarcinoma within the pancreatic head: a hypoenhancing mass (*purple arrows*) on the postcontrast late arterial phase (*A*) with high signal intensity (*B*) on DWI and low signal intensity (*C*) on the apparent diffusion coefficient (ADC) map indicating the mass restricts diffusion, a finding associated with tumors with densely packed cells restricting free movement of water molecules. MRI showing (*A*) hypoenhancing pancreatic tumor and (*B*) restricted diffusion (*C*) ADC.

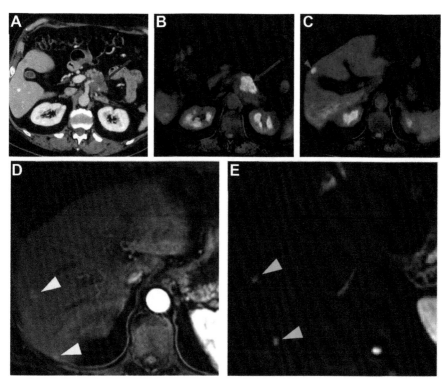

Fig. 6. Late arterial phase CT scan (*A*) demonstrates a low-attenuation pancreatic body mass with advanced locoregional invasion (*purple arrow*) and questionable lesion in the liver (*red arrowhead*). Subsequent PET/MR was acquired with fused PET/MR images of the pancreatic body (*B*) and liver (*C*) demonstrating avid FDG uptake associated with the pancreatic mass and liver lesion confirming a liver metastasis. Additional conventional MR images are routinely acquired with PET/MR with the late arterial postcontrast (*D*) and diffusion-weighed (*E*) sequences demonstrating subtle ring enhancing lesions (*yellow arrowheads*) in the right hepatic lobe with diffusion restriction (*blue arrowheads*) compatible with additional micrometastases; these micrometastases were not seen on diagnostic CT or PET images.

problematic in the elderly, in patients with significant comorbidities or deconditioning, and with patients receiving sedation or anxiolysis. The sensitivity of abdominal MRI to patient motion, both respiratory motion and general patient motion, is a limiting factor for MRI, although less motion-sensitive techniques are being developed.[9] Magnetic field strength of at least 1.5 T is preferred, which is a field strength readily available at most centers performing MRI examinations.[3]

Similar to CT scanning, dynamic postcontrast images demonstrate hypoenhancement of PDAC relative the normal pancreas (**Fig. 5**). Likewise, early postcontrast sequences are useful for analyzing the arterial anatomy. Late and delayed postcontrast images are helpful for examining venous relationships and detecting metastatic disease.[3]

DWI is an additional tool used in MRI for the evaluation of pancreatic cancer. DWI exploits the restriction of normal diffusion of water molecules in highly cellular or dense structures, including pancreatic tumors and liver metastases. Restricted diffusion is

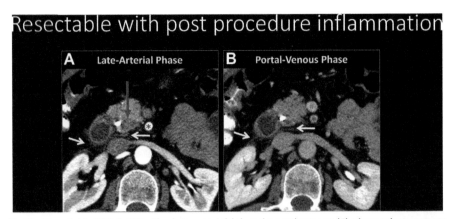

Fig. 7. Resectable PDAC. CT in the late arterial (*A*) and portal venous (*B*) phases demonstrate a low-attenuation mass completely confined to the pancreas with no tumor contact of the superior mesenteric artery (*red **) and vein (*blue #*) with primary tumor seen best on the arterial phase. Note a plastic endobiliary stent was placed before this staging CT scan with subtle peripancreatic and periduodenal fat stranding likely representing postplacement pancreatitis/inflammation (*yellow arrows*). Sometimes inflammation can be confused with extrapancreatic tumor extension and confound interpretation for accurate staging. Typically, the staging CT scan should be performed before stent placement to avoid this pitfall.

seen as a hyperintense signal on DWI and a correspondingly hypointense signal on the apparent diffusion coefficient map (see **Fig. 5**). The sensitivity and specificity of DWI for detecting both primary pancreatic tumors and liver metastases have been reported to be greater than 90%.[9,12,13]

Although not currently widely used, PET/MRI is being investigated for its usefulness in identifying locoregional lymph node metastases and distant metastatic disease in patients with pancreatic cancer.[9,14–17] PET/MRI may offer some advantages over

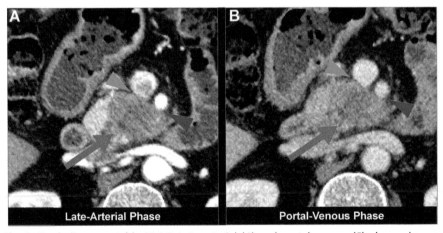

Fig. 8. Borderline resectable PDAC. Late arterial (*A*) and portal venous (*B*) phases demonstrate a large low-attenuation mass compatible with PDAC (*purple arrow*). The anterior margin of the tumor abuts (<180°) the posterior walls of the superior mesenteric artery (*red arrowhead*) and vein (*blue arrowhead*).

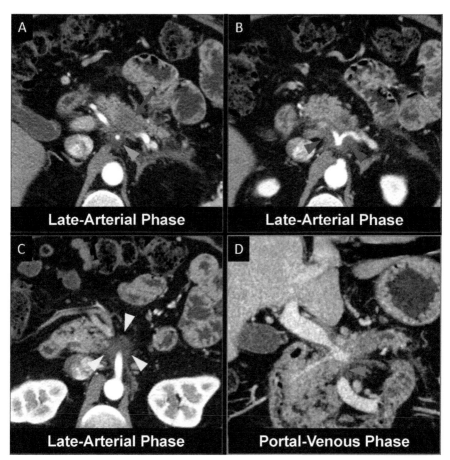

Fig. 9. Locally advanced PDAC. Late arterial phases (*A–C*) at several levels demonstrate a low-attenuation mass in the pancreatic body (*purple arrow*) with advanced locoregional extrapancreatic tumor extension with soft tissue encasing (>180°) the left gastric artery (*green arrowhead*), celiac bifurcation (*red arrowheads*), and superior mesenteric artery (*yellow arrowheads*). Portal venous phase coronal image (*D*) demonstrates the mass causing severe narrowing of the cephalad superior mesenteric vein with a "gap" below the portal–splenic–SMV venous confluence (*blue arrowhead*).

PET/CT scanning, including improved soft tissue contrast of MRI over CT scanning and highly accurate colocalization of PET tracer uptake with the anatomic MR images (**Fig. 6**). It also holds promise for assessing response to neoadjuvant therapy by combining the strengths of DWI and metabolic data.[9,15,18,19]

Initial Staging

The cornerstone of staging of PDAC is imaging. Either a CT scan or MRI can be used as discussed in the technique section, with a CT scan generally the preferred modality. A CT scan is preferred over other imaging modalities given its wide availability, superb spatial resolution, fast acquisition, and referring physicians' familiarity with its interpretation.[1–4] Although several societies publish staging criteria, including the TNM (tumor,

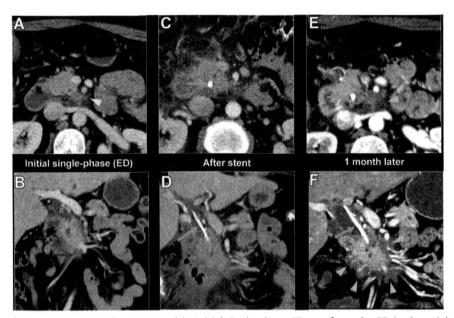

Fig. 10. Postintervention pancreatitis. Initial single-phase CT scan from the ED in the axial (*A*) and coronal (*B*) planes demonstrate a subtle uncinate process low-attenuation mass (*purple arrow*) with subtle extrapancreatic fat stranding (inflammation and/or tumor) possible abutting the superior mesenteric artery (*yellow arrowhead*). Note obstruction with dilation of the extrahepatic bile duct (*green B*). Before obtaining a dual-phase CT scan, the patient was emergently taken to endoscopy to relieve biliary obstruction with a plastic stent (*greed arrows*). A CT scan after biliary stenting in the axial (*C*) and coronal (*D*) planes demonstrated the subtle tumor in the uncinate process is not well-seen and there is extensive peripancreatic, periduodenal, and transverse mesocolonic inflammation (*red arrowheads*) compatible with postprocedure pancreatitis. 1 month later, a dual phase CT scan was acquired to complete staging. Axial (*E*) and coronal (*F*) images demonstrate the subtle uncinate process mass can be visible again, and there is now extensive peripancreatic soft tissue entrapping/encasing several superior mesenteric artery and vein branches (orange *arrowheads*). The soft tissue is likely post-pancreatitis inflammation, however, these findings are indeterminate by CT and confounds accurate staging.

node, metastasis) system of the American Joint Commission on Cancer, the most widely adopted staging system is from the National Comprehensive Cancer Network.[1,20,21] The National Comprehensive Cancer Network divides the initial stage of localized (nonmetastatic) pancreatic cancer into 3 surgical groups based on the lesion's relationship to the peripancreatic vasculature: resectable, borderline resectable, and locally advanced (**Figs. 7–9**). The previously mentioned societies continue to update their classification systems as surgical techniques evolve and outcomes improve, and it is therefore important for both radiologists and their clinical colleagues to be current with any revisions. In addition, institutional variations and modifications for both staging and management of pancreatic cancer exist, and it is important for the radiologist to be aware of institutional preferences. Imaging of the chest and pelvis are also generally performed for complete staging.

It is critical to obtain an initial staging dual-phase CT scan before any intervention is done or neoadjuvant therapy is started. Severe peripancreatic inflammation generated by biopsy, endoscopic retrograde cholangiopancreatography, and/or biliary stenting can obscure the tumor and tumor–vascular relationships on CT scans, thereby delaying accurate staging until the inflammation has subsided, which can be many weeks (**Fig. 10**). Milder degrees of inflammation can mimic tumor or desmoplasia and lead to inaccurate staging. In addition, peripancreatic edema, lymphatic congestion, and fibrosis induced by neoadjuvant chemoradiation can seem similar to tumor and lead to an overestimation of tumor size and vascular involvement.

Other imaging modalities can be used as adjuncts to initial staging with CT scanning. These techniques include endoscopic ultrasound examination, endoscopic retrograde cholangiopancreatography, PET, and MRI.[1,9] Endoscopic ultrasound examination is mostly used to provide more information on tumors that are occult on imaging (at the ampulla, for example) and for guidance for endoscopic biopsy. Endoscopic retrograde cholangiopancreatography is used in combination with stenting as a therapeutic method to relieve biliary obstruction. MRCP is used as a diagnostic tool to noninvasively evaluate the biliary and pancreatic ducts. PET/CT scanning is used to screen for metastatic disease in high-risk individuals.

Neoadjuvant Therapy

Neoadjuvant therapy is increasingly being used for treatment of PDAC. The rationale, indications, and use of neoadjuvant therapies are beyond the scope of this article. Simply, the goal of neoadjuvant therapy is to downstage the tumor, or at least increase the likelihood of a negative resection margin (R0 resection). A favorable response on imaging can be intuitively hopeful, because a pathologic response has been shown to increase disease-free survival; however, CT scanning is limited in its ability to accurately predict pathologic response or successful R0 resection.[22,23] In fact, even a positive response on a restaging CT scan cannot be correlated with pathologic response.[23] Furthermore, it is becoming more widely accepted that patients deemed borderline resectable can undergo surgery if imaging does not demonstrate disease

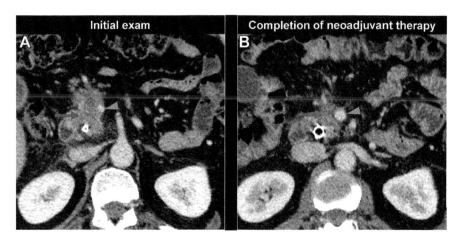

Fig. 11. Axial images in the portal venous phase at initial examination (*A*) and after completion of neoadjuvant therapy (*B*). Note the solid hypoenhancing mass (*purple arrows*) in the pancreatic head with extrapancreatic tumor encasing the superior mesenteric vein with severe narrowing (*blue arrowheads*). After completion of neoadjuvant therapy, there is reduction in size of the primary tumor, improved tumor–venous contact, and completely resolved vein narrowing. The patient subsequently underwent pancreatoduodenectomy (R0) with superior mesenteric vein resection and reconstruction with interposition vein graft.

progression over the course of neoadjuvant therapy,[1] and the R0 resection rate has been reported as high as 92% among patients with borderline or locally advanced disease after neoadjuvant therapy.[24]

There are several potential reasons for the discrepancy between CT findings and pathologic findings following neoadjuvant therapy.[22–25] A CT scan does not reliably differentiate infiltrative tumor from the desmoplastic reaction that may be induced in treated PDAC. Likewise, despite a tumor having actually decreased in size, a CT scan may demonstrate a stable lesion owing to the resultant replacement of tumor by peripancreatic inflammation, fibrosis, or lymphatic congestion being interpreted as tumor, particularly in patients receiving chemoradiation. In addition, patients with tumors in the head of the pancreas often need biliary interventions and stent placement, a potential source of infection and pancreatitis that can confound restaging on imaging. The retrospective observation that continued apparent tumor contact of the peripancreatic vasculature after neoadjuvant therapy is not necessarily associated with invasive disease and that overall survival after neoadjuvant therapy is similar between radiologic responders and nonresponders further highlights the limitations of imaging. Although a favorable imaging response to treatment can be reassuring, in cases where imaging demonstrates a seeming lack of response, knowing that a CT scan is limited in its ability to differentiate tumor from treatment-related changes is an important consideration for the oncologic care team (**Fig. 11**).

Given the limitations of CT scans to accurately assess response to neoadjuvant therapy, other imaging techniques have been investigated and may hold promise such as PET scans, CT texture analysis, and MRI with DWI. For example, patients with a metabolic response on PET scans were more likely to have a pathologic response seen at the time of surgery.[19] CT texture analysis is a technique that evaluates spatial variation in voxel intensities within a CT image to quantify the perceived texture of an image. Changes in specific CT textural features, which often go unnoticed to the naked eye, may reflect pathologic tumor response.[9,26,27] In addition,

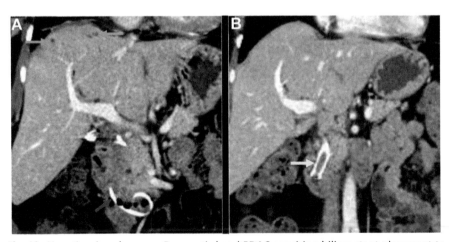

Fig. 12. Hepatic microabscesses. Pancreatic head PDAC requiring biliary stent placement to relieve biliary obstruction. Coronal image (*A*) after plastic endobiliary stent placement (*pink arrow*) demonstrates tiny clustered hypoattenuating lesions in the liver dome (*green arrows*). Follow-up coronal image 20 days later (*B*) after antibiotics and exchange of the plastic stent for a more durable metallic stent (*yellow arrow*) demonstrates resolution of the liver dome microabscesses.

several studies have shown changes in DWI metrics on MRI to be associated with histologic response.[28] The investigation of these and other imaging methods are ongoing.

Indeterminate Liver Lesions

A CT scan is the preferred method for the initial staging of pancreatic cancer given its superiority in demonstrating vascular relationships. However, a CT scan is limited in its ability to detect metastatic disease. Adjuncts to CT scanning are often needed owing to a high incidence of patients presenting with liver lesions at the time of diagnosis, as high as 41% in a recent study.[29] Of those patients with liver lesions, 72% were considered indeterminate on a CT scan.

A challenge for CT scanning in the staging of pancreatic cancer is characterizing small liver lesions, particularly those less than 1.5 cm. Although additional imaging studies can be performed including MRI, PET, or ultrasound examination, the additional costs of these tests may not be justified, because small indeterminate lesions often remain indeterminate despite additional attempts at characterization.[29]

To better serve patients in a cost-effective and timely manner, a stratification system has been proposed to help identify which patients should undergo an additional workup. A retrospective analysis found that the radiologist stratifying "indeterminate" liver lesions based on objective imaging features into categories of "indeterminate, probably benign" or "indeterminate, possibly malignant" was a robust method for determining which lesions could be observed versus requiring additional follow-up tests. The negative predictive value was 94% for those findings placed into the "indeterminate, probably benign" category. In contrast, if a lesion was labeled "indeterminate, possibly malignant," there was an approximately 30% chance of actually representing metastatic disease.[29]

MRI can be helpful for characterizing indeterminate liver lesions found on a CT scan.[1,3,30] Because common benign liver lesions, such as cysts, hemangiomas, and focal nodular hyperplasia, have characteristic features on MRI, they can be identified reliably and differentiated from metastases. Lesions not having features of typical benign lesions should be viewed with suspicion. As with CT and PET scanning, differentiation of small liver metastases from microabscesses secondary to biliary stent manipulation is exceedingly difficult with MRI owing to overlapping imaging features and confident differentiation of these entities may not be possible by imaging (**Fig. 12**).

A PET/CT scan can be useful for confirming suspected liver metastases, particularly in lesions greater than 1 cm. A PET/CT scan is limited for the characterization of lesions less than 1 cm, because sensitivity for detection of subcentimeter liver metastases by PET scan is limited.[14] Furthermore, hypermetabolic activity can be seen in both liver metastases and microabscesses, and differentiation of these 2 entities can be difficult, particularly in subcentimeter lesions.

REPORTING

Structured radiology reporting has gained widespread adaptation by more clearly and effectively communicating crucial information required for consistent staging and treatment planning.[4,31] Use of template radiology reports has been shown to provide more complete and accurate staging of PDAC than free-text dictation, because it ensures that all the critical vascular relationships and tumor details are described and provides consistent use of terminology.[1,4,31,32] Furthermore, data mining for both research and quality assurance is better with structured reports. For these reasons,

Medical College of Wisconsin – Pancreatic Cancer Staging

Examination(s):
[1. CT angiography abdomen with IV contrast.]
2. CT pelvis with IV contrast.]

Clinical Information: [Pancreatic mass. Initial staging.]

Comparison: [None.]

Technique:
IV contrast: [125] mL [Omnipaque 350].
Oral contrast: [None].
3D Imaging: [Multiplanar MIP, curved planar, and 3D volume rendered images are created by the 3D lab.]
Technical comments: [Dual-phase imaging of the abdomen.]
Dose reduction. [This CT exam was performed using one or more of the following dose-reduction techniques: Automated exposure control, adjustment of the mA and/or kV according to patient size, and/or use of iterative reconstruction technique.]

Findings:

PANCREAS

Primary tumor: [[AP x transvers x craniocaudal]] cm [low-attenuation] mass in the [***] [series]), image # []].

Pancreatic duct: [Dilated] [] mm.

[No other pancreatic mass is identified. The pancreas is otherwise normal.]

MESENTERIC ARTERIES

Arterial anatomy: [Normal (Type I).]

Arterial tumor abutment or encasement:

Celiac, common/proper hepatic, proximal splenic, left gastric and gastroduodenal arteries: [None | Abutment (less than or equal to 180 degrees) | Encasement (greater than 180 degrees).]

Superior mesenteric artery: [None | Abutment (less than or equal to 180 degrees) | Encasement (greater than 180 degrees).]

Other findings: [NONE or Tumor abutment or encasement of additional arteries (i.e., IPDA, GDA, jejunal, middle colic, or ileocolic branches).]

MESENTERIC VEINS

Venous anatomy:

Superior mesenteric vein (SMV) 1st jejunal branch: [posterior to SMA.]

Inferior mesenteric vein (IMV) drains into the SMV inferior to the [portosplenic confluence.]

Venous tumor abutment or encasement:

SMV-PV-splenic vein confluence: [None | Abutment (less than or equal to 180 degrees) | Encasement (greater than 180 degrees).]

First jejunal vein branch: [None | Abutment (less than or equal to 180 degrees) | Encasement (greater than 180 degrees.]

SMV, PV, or segmental SMV-PV occlusion: [None.]

Other findings: [NONE or Tumor abutment or encasement of jejunal, middle colic, gastroepiploic, or ileal branches of the SMV or Long/short segment (approximately x cm) of tumor free SMV inferior (caudal) to diseased segment.]

Portal venous system: [Normal and patent.]

Inferior vena cava (IVC): [Normal.]

HEPATOBILIARY SYSTEM

Focal liver lesions: [None.]

Biliary tree: [No endobiliary stent]. [No intrahepatic or extrahepatic biliary dilatation.] CBD [] mm.

Gallbladder: [Present.]

LOCOREGIONAL SPREAD

Lymph nodes: [No adenopathy.]

Peritoneum: [Negative. No nodularity or thickening.]

Omentum: [Negative. No nodularity or thickening.]

Ascites: [None.]

OTHER FINDINGS

Stomach, small bowel, and large bowel: [Normal wall thickness, caliber, and enhancement.]

Genitourinary system: [Normal.]

Adrenal glands: [Normal.]

Spleen: [Normal.]

Lower chest: [Normal.]

Bones: [No significant lesion].

Impression:
1. Pancreatic [head] mass measuring [] cm consistent with [pancreatic adenocarcinoma].
2. [No metastatic disease.]
3. [No adenopathy.]
4. [No arterial or venous abutment or encasement.]
5. [Other impression statements]

Fig. 13. Standardized radiology structured reporting (SR) templated used at the Medical College of Wisconsin. SRs can be programmed within radiology voice recognition dictation systems for easier use.

it is highly recommended that initial staging and preoperative examinations are read and reported using a structured report.[4,31] A modified structured report based on the Society of Abdominal Radiology's available template[4] was collaboratively created between radiology, surgical oncology, hematology–oncology, gastroenterology, and radiation oncology at our intuition and is used consistently for every staging examination (**Fig. 13**).

DISCLOSURE

The authors have nothing to disclose.

REFERENCES

1. Kulkarni NM, Soloff Ev, Tolat PP, et al. White paper on pancreatic ductal adenocarcinoma from society of abdominal radiology's disease-focused panel for pancreatic ductal adenocarcinoma: Part I, AJCC staging system, NCCN guidelines, and borderline resectable disease. Abdom Radiol 2020;45(3):716–28.
2. Callery MP, Chang KJ, Fishman EK, et al. Pretreatment assessment of resectable and borderline resectable pancreatic cancer: expert consensus statement. Ann Surg Oncol 2009;16:1727–33.
3. Kulkarni NM, Hough DM, Tolat PP, et al. Pancreatic adenocarcinoma: cross-sectional imaging techniques. Abdom Radiol 2018;43(2):253–63.
4. Al-Hawary MM, Francis IR, Chari ST, et al. Pancreatic ductal adenocarcinoma radiology reporting template: consensus statement of the society of abdominal radiology and the American Pancreatic Association. Radiology 2014;270(1):248–60.
5. Fukukura Y, Takumi K, Kamiyama T, et al. Pancreatic adenocarcinoma: a comparison of automatic bolus tracking and empirical scan delay. Abdom Imaging 2010;35(5):548–55.
6. Foley WD, Kerimoglu U. Abdominal MDCT: liver, pancreas, and biliary tract. Semin Ultrasound CT MRI 2004;25(2):122–44.
7. Morgan DE. Dual-energy CT of the abdomen. Abdom Imaging 2014;39(1):108–34.
8. Kulkarni NM, Pinho DF, Kambadakone AR, et al. Emerging technologies in CT- radiation dose reduction and dual-energy CT. Semin Roentgenol 2013;48(3):192–202.
9. Kulkarni NM, Mannelli L, Zins M, et al. White paper on pancreatic ductal adenocarcinoma from society of abdominal radiology's disease-focused panel for pancreatic ductal adenocarcinoma: Part II, update on imaging techniques and screening of pancreatic cancer in high-risk individuals. Abdom Radiol 2020;45(3):729–42.
10. Ichikawa T, Mehmet Erturk S, Sou H, et al. MDCT of pancreatic adenocarcinoma MDCT of pancreatic adenocarcinoma: optimal imaging phases and multiplanar reformatted imaging. AJR Am J Roentgenol 2006;187. https://doi.org/10.2214/AJR.05.1031.
11. O'Neill E, Hammond N, Miller FH. MR imaging of the pancreas. Radiol Clin North Am 2014;52(4):757–77.
12. Marion-Audibert AM, Vullierme MP, Ronot M, et al. Routine MRI with DWI sequences to detect liver metastases in patients with potentially resectable pancreatic ductal carcinoma and normal liver CT: a prospective multicenter study. AJR Am J Roentgenol 2018;211(5):W217–25.

13. Ichikawa T, Erturk SM, Motosugi U, et al. High-b value diffusion-weighted MRI for detecting pancreatic adenocarcinoma: preliminary results. AJR Am J Roentgenol 2007;188(2):409–14.
14. Yeh R, Dercle L, Garg I, et al. The role of 18F-FDG PET/CT and PET/MRI in pancreatic ductal adenocarcinoma. Abdom Radiol 2018;43(2):415–34.
15. Mallak N, Hope TA, Guimaraes AR. PET/MR imaging of the pancreas. Magn Reson Imaging Clin North Am 2018;26(3):345–62.
16. Paspulati RM, Gupta A. PET/MR imaging in cancers of the gastrointestinal tract. PET Clin 2016;11(4):403–23.
17. Chen B bin, Tien YW, Chang MC, et al. Multiparametric PET/MR imaging biomarkers are associated with overall survival in patients with pancreatic cancer. Eur J Nucl Med Mol Imaging 2018;45(7):1205–17.
18. Wang ZJ, Behr S, Consunji Mv, et al. Early response assessment in pancreatic ductal adenocarcinoma through integrated PET/MRI. AJR Am J Roentgenol 2018;211(5):1010–9.
19. Panda A, Garg I, Truty MJ, et al. Borderline resectable and locally advanced pancreas cancer: FDG PET/MRI and CT tumor metrics for assessment of neoadjuvant therapy pathologic response and prediction of survival. AJR Am J Roentgenol 2020. https://doi.org/10.2214/ajr.20.24567.
20. Amin MB, editor. AJCC cancer staging manual. 8th edition. Chicago, IL, USA: Springer International Publishing; 2017.
21. NCCN Clinical Practice Guidelines in Oncology (NCCN Guidelines) Version 2.2019 - Pancreatic Adenocarcinoma.; 2018.
22. Wagner M, Antunes C, Pietrasz D, et al. CT evaluation after neoadjuvant FOLFIRINOX chemotherapy for borderline and locally advanced pancreatic adenocarcinoma. Eur Radiol 2017;27(7):3104–16.
23. Xia BT, Fu B, Wang J, et al. Does radiologic response correlate to pathologic response in patients undergoing neoadjuvant therapy for borderline resectable pancreatic malignancy? J Surg Oncol 2017;115(4):376–83.
24. Ferrone CR, Marchegiani G, Hong TS, et al. Radiological and surgical implications of neoadjuvant treatment with FOLFIRINOX for locally advanced and borderline resectable pancreatic cancer. Ann Surg 2015;261:12–7.
25. Cassinotto C, Cortade J, Belleannée G, et al. An evaluation of the accuracy of CT when determining resectability of pancreatic head adenocarcinoma after neoadjuvant treatment. Eur J Radiol 2013;82(4):589–93.
26. Guo C, Zhuge X, Wang Z, et al. Textural analysis on contrast-enhanced CT in pancreatic neuroendocrine neoplasms: association with WHO grade. Abdom Radiol 2019;44(2):576–85.
27. Lubner MG, Smith AD, Sandrasegaran K, et al. CT texture analysis: definitions, applications, biologic correlates, and challenges. Radiographics 2017;37(5):1483–503.
28. Dalah E, Erickson B, Oshima K, et al. Correlation of ADC with pathological treatment response for radiation therapy of pancreatic cancer. Translational Oncol 2018;11(2):391–8.
29. Bhalla M, Aldakkak M, Kulkarni NM, et al. Characterizing indeterminate liver lesions in patients with localized pancreatic cancer at the time of diagnosis. Abdom Radiol 2018;43(2):351–63.
30. Raman SP, Horton KM, Fishman EK. Multimodality imaging of pancreatic cancer-computed tomography, magnetic resonance imaging, and positron emission tomography. Cancer J (United States) 2012;18(6):511–22.

31. Brook OR, Brook A, Vollmer CM, et al. Structured reporting of multiphasic CT for pancreatic cancer: Potential effect on staging and surgical planning. Radiology 2015;274(2):464–72.
32. Marcal LP, Fox PS, Evans DB, et al. Analysis of free-form radiology dictations for completeness and clarity for pancreatic cancer staging. Abdom Imaging 2015; 40(7):2391–7.

Advanced Endoscopic Techniques for the Diagnosis of Pancreatic Cancer and Management of Biliary and GastricOutlet Obstruction

Yousuke Nakai, MD[a], Zachary Smith, MD[b],
Kenneth J. Chang, MD[c],
Kulwinder S. Dua, MD, DMSc, FRCP (L), FRCP (E), FACP, MASGE[b],*

KEYWORDS

- Endoscopic retrograde cholangiopancreatography • Endoscopic ultrasonography
- Gastric outlet obstruction • Malignant biliary obstruction • Pancreatic cancer
- Stents

KEY POINTS

- Endoscopic ultrasound examination plays an important role in detection, tissue acquisition, and staging of pancreatic cancer.
- Endoscopic retrograde cholangiopancreatography with biliary metal stent placement is the mainstay of palliation of malignant biliary obstruction but endoscopic ultrasound-guided biliary drainage can also be a treatment option.
- For patients with resectable pancreatic cancer, endoscopic retrograde cholangiopancreatography with biliary stenting should be avoided if early surgery is being planned.
- Metal biliary stents provide durable biliary drainage and can safely be placed in those where surgery is going to be delayed (example, neoadjuvant therapy).
- Enteral stenting is often selected for palliation of gastric outlet obstruction because of its less invasiveness but the rate of recurrent symptoms is higher than surgical gastrojejunostomy. Endoscopic ultrasound-guided gastrojejunostomy can be considered and initial outcomes have been promising.

[a] Department of Endoscopy and Endoscopic Surgery, The University of Tokyo Hospital, 7-3-1, Hongo, Bunkyo-ku, Tokyo, Japan; [b] Division of Gastroenterology and Hepatology, Medical College of Wisconsin, 9200, West Wisconsin Avenue, Milwaukee, WI, USA; [c] Division of Gastroenterology and Hepatology, Digestive Health Institute, University of California, Irvine, 101 The City Drive, Building 22C, Orange, CA, USA
* Corresponding author. Division of Gastroenterology and Hepatology, Medical College of Wisconsin, 9200, West Wisconsin Avenue, Milwaukee, WI.
E-mail address: kdua@mcw.edu

Surg Oncol Clin N Am 30 (2021) 639–656
https://doi.org/10.1016/j.soc.2021.06.005

INTRODUCTION

Pancreatic cancer is the fourth leading cause of cancer deaths in the United States, with an estimated of 55,600 new cases and 47,050 deaths in 2020.[1] The early diagnosis of pancreatic cancer is still difficult, and its prognosis is poor with a 5-year survival rate of 9% in all cases and 3% in cases with metastatic diseases. Endoscopic ultrasound examination (EUS) and endoscopic retrograde cholangiopancreatography (ERCP) are 2 endoscopic procedures used in the diagnosis and management of pancreatic cancer. The role of endoscopy is both diagnostic with detection, staging and tissue acquisition, as well as therapeutic with palliation of malignant biliary obstruction (MBO) and gastric outlet obstruction (GOO). Although EUS-guided ablation or injection for pancreatic cancer has been of emerging interest,[2] it is still considered experimental. In this article, we discuss the endoscopic diagnosis of pancreatic cancer and endoscopic palliation of MBO and GOO.

DIAGNOSIS OF PANCREATIC CANCER
Detection

A pancreatic protocol computed tomography (CT) scan is the first step for detection and diagnosis when there is a clinical suspicion of pancreatic cancer. Despite clinical suspicion, if a mass is not seen on the CT scan, EUS examination should be considered because it has better sensitivity than a CT scan in identifying lesions smaller than 1 cm. In a systematic review including 19 studies by Kitano and colleagues,[3] EUS examination provides a higher sensitivity of 94% as compared with 74% by CT scan. However, 11 of the studies analyzed were conducted in the 1990s and the sensitivity of CT scan has significantly improved since then by the wide spread use of multidetector (≥64 slices) CT scans with a pancreatic protocol. However, it is well-known that the spatial resolution is better with EUS examination and a systematic review of 206 cases with indeterminate multidetector CT scan showed that EUS examination detected a mass in 70% with a mean size 21 mm.[4] Thus, although the diagnostic yield of EUS examination is more operator dependent than a CT scan, EUS examination has an advantage of detecting small pancreatic masses (**Fig. 1**).

Staging

It should be noted that the treatment strategy for pancreatic cancer has evolved to include the adoption of neoadjuvant treatment. Clinical staging for treatment selection

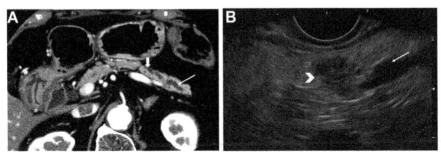

CT Scan   EUS Scan

Fig. 1. (*A*) Computed tomography (CT) scan showed pancreatic duct dilation (*arrow*) in the tail with a cut-off in the body (*broad arrow*), but no mass was seen. (*B*) Endoscopic ultrasound (EUS) examination of the same patient showed a 10-mm irregular mass (*arrowhead*) at the caliber change of the pancreatic duct.

used to be dichotomized to resectable versus nonresectable lesions, but now the staging is further segmented into resectable, borderline resectable, and nonresectable. Clinical staging is mainly determined by the extent of local vascular involvement and the presence of distant metastases.

EUS examination can be used to detect the relationship of the tumor to adjacent vascular structures. In a systematic review,[5] the sensitivity of EUS examination and CT scans to detect tumor contact with adjacent vasculature was 72% and 63%, and specificity was 89% and 92%, respectively. Interestingly, when analyzed in 3 different time periods (1993–2009, 2000–2005, and 2006–2013), the diagnostic yield defined by the area under the curve decreased in EUS area under the curve from 0.9563 in the first period to 0.8539 in the last period. Meanwhile, area under the curve of CT scans increased from 0.8974 in the first period to 0.9769 in the last period, which may be attributed to both the advancing technology of CT scanners and the initial overestimation and enthusiasm of EUS diagnosis in those early days. The overall quality of studies included in the analysis was not high and the heterogeneity between studies hindered a solid conclusion. Based on recent criteria for resectability by National Comprehensive Cancer Network guidelines,[6] resectability status is determined not only by the presence of vascular contact, but the circumferential extent of vascular contact is used to differentiate resectable, borderline resectable, and locally advanced diseases. Reproducibility of the degree of vascular contact is better with a pancreatic protocol CT scan, rather than EUS examination. Furthermore, a common strategy is to offer neoadjuvant treatment even to patients with resectable lesions. In a recent randomized controlled trial (RCT) of resectable pancreatic cancer (Prep-02/JSAP-05),[7] neoadjuvant chemotherapy demonstrated longer overall survival with a hazard ratio of 0.72 (P = .015). Thus, we are moving toward neoadjuvant treatment in resectable and borderline resectable pancreatic cancers, and the role of detailed staging at the time of diagnosis might decrease because most patients will undergo neoadjuvant treatment, regardless of the presence of vascular invasion. Patient selection for surgical resection after neoadjuvant treatment is currently under investigation but it is still unclear whether imaging modalities such as CT scan and EUS examination, or biomarkers such as carbohydrate antigen 19-9, can better predict resectability and prognosis after neoadjuvant treatment.

For detection of distant metastasis, a CT scan or PET scan is generally used, but EUS examination can also detect distant metastases, that is, nonregional lymph nodes, liver metastases, and peritoneal dissemination. Kurita and colleagues[8] compared the diagnostic yield of EUS examination with fine needle aspiration (EUS-FNA) and PET-CT scan to detect nonregional lymph node metastases. The sensitivity of EUS-FNA and PET-CT scan was 96.7% and 53.3%, respectively (P<.001), and unnecessary laparotomy was avoided in 15.4% of patients with para-aortic lymph node. Small liver lesions can be detected by EUS examination as well. EUS examination detected liver lesions in 8.5% of patients by B-mode images,[9] although EUS visualization of the liver is limited mainly to the left lobe. More recently, the usefulness of Kupffer phase imaging of contrast-enhanced harmonic EUS examination is reported in detecting small liver lesions. The diagnostic accuracy of contrast-enhanced CT scans, B-mode EUS examination, and contrast-enhanced harmonic EUS examination was 90.6%, 93.4%, and 98.4%, respectively, and only contrast-enhanced harmonic EUS examination can detect small (<10 mm) liver lesions in 2.1% of cases.[10] Finally, EUS examination can also diagnosis carcinomatosis even in patients with no or minimal ascites; that is, 29.6% with ascites and in 3.7% without ascites. Among 106 cases with a resectable lesion on CT scan, EUS examination detected ascites in 18 cases and 4 of them had carcinomatosis.[11] Thus, in the era of neoadjuvant treatment, the value of EUS staging in pancreatic cancer is shifting from evaluation of local vascular invasion to detection of distant metastases to better stratify patients who would benefit from resection.

Tissue Acquisition

EUS-FNA for pancreatic masses was first reported in the early 1990s[12,13] and is now established as the standard tissue acquisition method. The sensitivity and specificity of EUS-FNA for pancreatic masses were 85% to 91% and 96% to 98%, respectively.[3] Potential adverse events are pain, pancreatitis, and bleeding, and the adverse event rate was 2.4% in prospective studies.[14] EUS-guided fine needle biopsy (EUS-FNB), which was developed to improve the diagnostic yield of EUS-FNA, is now widely used in clinical practice. Currently, several FNB needles are commercially available such as a reverse or forward bevel needle,[15–17] a Franseen needle,[18] and a fork-tip needle.[19] There have been numerous, well-done, prospective clinical trials comparing FNA to FNB needles. Because the diagnostic yield of EUS-FNA is so high, it has been difficult to prove diagnostic superiority of FNB to FNA.[20] One of the clear cut advantage of EUS-FNB over EUS-FNA is the ability to determine specimen adequacy by visual inspection of the gross specimen, and thereby decrease the number of passes needed for diagnosis, especially in the absence of rapid onsite evaluation.[21]

Although there is certainly an emerging trend moving from FNA to FNB, ultimately the details of the tissue acquisition will depend on what the specimen will be used for in the future. The type of needle used, the technique used, and the tissue handling that ensues should be tailored toward the type of specimen needed and the expertise of the pathologist or cytologist. The tissue specimen can be viewed as a spectrum, from cytology (single cells), to cell block, to fragmented core tissue, to histologically intact core tissue. Although in an ideal scenario 1 needle and technique would be able to provide the entire spectrum of specimens, from cytology to histologically using intact core tissue, that may not yet be possible.

There may be clinical situations where a high cytologic yield is important; for example, to make a cancer diagnosis by rapid staining and determine whether a metal versus plastic biliary stent should be placed during the same session. In addition, providing the patient with an immediate diagnosis allows the opportunity for more specific postprocedure discussion and management plans. However, other clinical situations call for an abundance of tissue, whether histologically intact or not. Recent studies have shown that EUS-FNB provides adequate specimen for genome profiling for pancreatic cancer.[22] Genomic profiling is gaining more attention even in pancreatic cancer. In the National Comprehensive Cancer Network guidelines,[6] gene profiling of the tumor tissue in addition to germline testing is recommended in metastatic pancreatic cancer. Even though the proportion of patients who could receive targeted treatment after genome profiling is limited in pancreatic cancer, those who can receive targeted treatment gain survival benefits and the recent development of gene-specific treatments are a harbinger for more precision medicine treatment options in the future. Because EUS-guided tissue acquisition provides the chance to obtain tissue specimen in patients who would not undergo surgical resection, EUS-FNB is recommended in patients with unresectable pancreatic cancer for possible genomic profiling.

ERCP with pancreatic juice cytology was also used to diagnose pancreatic cancer in the past.[23] However, it is not routinely performed owing to its low sensitivity and high adverse event rate, especially post-ERCP pancreatitis. Of note, the novel technique called SPACE (serial pancreatic juice aspiration cytologic examination) is reported to diagnose early pancreatic cancer from Japan.[24–26]

Tumor seeding can occur after EUS-FNA and is of concern in cases with resectable pancreatic cancer. In the body and tail of pancreas, the needle tract of the gastric wall is not resected and recurrence owing to needle tract seeding can occur even after curative resection. In a large scale data of the linked Surveillance, Epidemiology, and End Results–Medicare, preoperative EUS-FNA did not impair survival.[27] However, in a recent Japanese multicenter retrospective study of 301 resected pancreatic cancer,[28] although recurrence-free survival and overall survival did not differ significantly with and without EUS-FNA, the rate of needle tract seeding after EUS-FNA was as high as 3.4%, which is higher than previously expected.

ENDOSCOPIC MANAGEMENT OF BILIARY OBSTRUCTION

Pancreatic cancer, especially in the head of pancreas, is often complicated by MBO. MBO can lead to jaundice and itching although spontaneous cholangitis is rare. Surgical choledochojejunostomy or percutaneous transhepatic biliary drainage (PTBD) used to be performed for biliary decompression but was associated with high morbidity and mortality. Endoscopic transpapillary biliary drainage via ERCP was introduced as a less invasive alternative. In an RCT by Speer and colleagues,[29] endoscopic biliary drainage (EBD) was shown to provide faster and effective resolution of jaundice with less mortality than PTBD. Later, Smith and colleagues[30] compared EBD and surgical bypass and EBD showed similar efficacy with less morbidity. EBD has now become the standard of care for those requiring biliary drainage owing to pancreatic cancer.

For EBD, 2 types of stents are available: plastic and metal. Self-expandable metal stents, with their larger diameter (usually 10 mm), were shown to provide longer stent patency than plastic stents,[31] but stent occlusion by tumor ingrowth through the stent mesh can occur in uncovered metal stents. To prevent tumor ingrowth, covered metal stents were developed (**Fig. 2**). Although some RCTs[32,33] demonstrated the superiority of covered metal stents over uncovered metal stents, the data are conflicting. A recent meta-analysis[34] showed that the hazard ratio for stent failure was 0.68, favoring covered metal stents, but the difference was not statistically significant. Although tumor ingrowth was less common (odds ratio, 0.21) with covered metal stents, stent migration (odds ratio, 5.11) and sludge formation (odds ratio, 2.46) were more common with covered metal stents. Although covered metal stents are believed to increase the risks of cholecystitis or pancreatitis by covering the orifice of the cystic duct or pancreatic duct, respectively, there were no significant differences in the rates of procedure-related adverse events. Covered metal stents are more expensive than uncovered stents. Although not yet approved by the US Food and Drug Administration for removable indication for MBO, covered metal stents can potentially be removed, unlike uncovered metal stents that get embedded with tissue ingrowth. Currently, there is no consensus regarding the use of covered or uncovered metal stents in MBO, although one would prefer to place a plastic or a covered metal stent if the diagnosis is not certain.

In cases with resectable pancreatic cancer, the role of preoperative biliary drainage is controversial. Studies have shown that postoperative infectious complications increase by preoperative biliary drainage. A RCT[35] was conducted comparing early surgery with or without preoperative biliary drainage in patients with resectable pancreatic cancer with biliary obstruction. In this study, preoperative biliary drainage increased serious perioperative complications (39% vs 74%) and the investigators concluded that routine preoperative biliary drainage should not be recommended in patients going for early surgery. However, the study was criticized for the use of

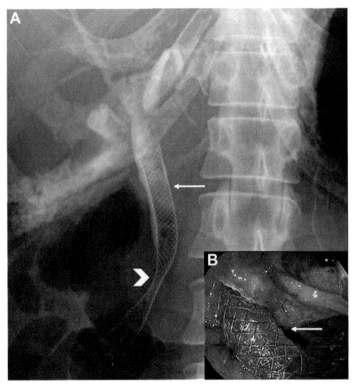

Fig. 2. Fluoroscopic (*A*) and endoscopic (*B*) views of a covered metal stent (*arrow*) for distal malignant biliary stricture (*arrowhead*).

preoperative plastic biliary stents,[36] which increased the rate of preoperative cholangitis. Moreover, the ERCP failure rate for preoperative drainage was higher than one would have expected, and these patients then required percutaneous drainage. The study group later reported the clinical outcomes of covered metal stents as preoperative biliary drainage and covered metal stents yielded better outcomes than plastic stents, but did not decrease perioperative complications when compared with early surgery without biliary drainage.[37]

Despite these study outcomes, in clinical practice, it is not always possible to perform surgery within 2 weeks of diagnosis of resectable pancreatic cancer, even at high-volume centers, and preoperative biliary drainage is often performed when surgery is delayed. Furthermore, as described elsewhere in this article, neoadjuvant treatment is being increasingly used and durable biliary drainage is mandatory to facilitate and maintain normal liver functions to allow for the administration of chemotherapy. Thus, the current debate is shifting from the necessity of preoperative biliary drainage to the stent selection for preoperative biliary drainage during neoadjuvant treatment. Many studies[38–42] have shown metal stents as preoperative biliary drainage are safe and effective and do not significantly affect surgical outcomes or interfere with surgery. In a study on 49 patients, plastic stents used during neoadjuvant therapy were associated frequent cholangitis, hospital admissions, and interruption of neoadjuvant therapy in around 55% of patients.[43] Hence, metal stents are preferable and it is not necessary to remove the stent before surgery as long as a "short" metal stent is placed so as to bridge the distal biliary obstruction and not reach up to the hilum of the liver.[41,42] Moreover, a recent RCT demonstrated that both covered and uncovered metal stents can be used in the neoadjuvant setting.[44] Thus, in cases with MBO owing to pancreatic cancer, either a covered or uncovered metal stent can be used as biliary drainage regardless of resectability. If the diagnosis is uncertain or rapid onsite evaluation of EUS-guided FNA/FNB is not available, one can consider placing a fully covered metal stent that potentially can be removed if required.

EUS-guided biliary drainage (EUS-BD) was recently reported as an alternative to endoscopic transpapillary biliary drainage. In this approach, biliary access is achieved by either puncturing the left intrahepatic bile ducts through the gastric wall or the common hepatic duct from the duodenal bulb with EUS guidance. A guidewire is then passed in the biliary duct, over which an expandable metal stent is placed (hepatico-gastrostomy or choledochoduodenostomy, respectively), or a the guidewire is advanced into the duodenum via the major papilla and a rendezvous procedure performed. EUS-BD was first reported in 2001 as a salvage technique after failed ERCP.[45] PTBD has been used as a salvage technique after failed ERCP, but EUS-BD is preferred to PTBD, with a higher clinical success rate and fewer adverse events when performed by experts.[46] In pancreatic cancer, combined MBO and GOO is often encountered and result in failed ERCP because GOO generally involves the second part of the duodenum and transpapillary biliary access is technically difficult or impossible.[47] Transpapillary stenting is prone to duodenobiliary reflux in cases with GOO and duodenal stenting[48–50] and EUS-BD can provide better stent patency.[51] Diversion of biliary drainage by EUS-guided hepaticogastrostomy is useful in combination with enteral stenting for combined MBO and GOO (**Fig. 3**).[52,53]

Recently, EUS-BD for MBO as a primary biliary drainage approach instead of ERCP is increasingly being considered. Three RCTs[54–56] were reported and although each of them was not powered to demonstrate the superiority of one over the other, EUS-BD was comparable with ERCP in terms of safety and patency when performed by experts. In addition, EUS-BD has the advantage of avoiding post-ERCP pancreatitis and may play a central role once dedicated devices such as a EUS-BD dedicated lumen-apposing metal stents[57] are available.

ENDOSCOPIC MANAGEMENT OF GASTRIC OUTLET OBSTRUCTION

Obstruction can occur in the setting of pancreatic cancer either before or after surgical resection. In patients with native anatomy, this blockage is commonly owing to a tumor-related obstruction. In patients who have undergone pancreaticoduodenectomy, intestinal obstruction can occur at several points. Alimentary obstruction can occur within the afferent or efferent loop or at the level of the gastrojejunostomy. Gastrojejunostomy obstructions, albeit very rare, are usually caused by stomal ulceration and stricturing and can be managed with acid suppression and endoscopic balloon dilation as needed. Efferent loop obstructions, also a rare phenomenon, are typically owing to internal hernias or adhesions, and there is little role for endoscopic therapy in these circumstances. The other point of postoperative intestinal obstruction is within the afferent limb, resulting in so-called afferent limb syndrome. Afferent limb syndrome most commonly results from radiation enteropathy or disease recurrence.

Preoperative Gastric Outlet Obstruction

Before surgical resection, malignant pancreatic tumors in the head, uncinate process, and less commonly, the neck, can cause GOO in approximately 15% of patients.[58] The most common symptoms of malignant GOO include abdominal pain and fullness, early satiety, vomiting, and heartburn or acid reflux. Surgical bypass remains a

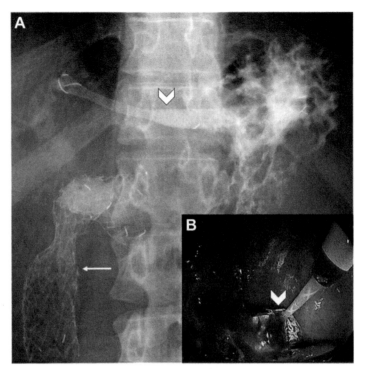

Fig. 3. (*A*) EUS-guided hepaticogastrostomy (*arrowhead*) and enteral stent (*arrow*) for combined MBO and GOO. (*B*) Endoscopic view of the stomach shows bile flowing through the stent that was used to create a hepaticogastrostomy (*arrowhead*).

mainstay within the treatment armamentarium for these patients. This condition may be especially true for patients with locally advanced disease who are surgically fit to undergo a laparoscopic bypass operation. Several studies have demonstrated greater durability of gastric decompression and lower reintervention rates with surgical bypass compared with enteral stenting.[59–61] For patients in whom an endoscopic approach is favored, there are several techniques available to achieve satisfactory decompression.

Percutaneous Endoscopic Gastroenterostomy Tubes

Although not a common first-line choice, percutaneous gastroenterostomy (GE) tubes still have a role in select circumstances where the enteral part of the tube is used to provide nutrition and the gastric part to decompress the stomach. In these circumstances, a larger bore, typically 24F to 28F, gastrostomy tube is placed in the typical endoscopic fashion. Using various techniques,[62–64] a deep enteral feeding tube is then inserted through the gastrostomy tube, over a previously placed guidewire, and into the small bowel distal to the obstruction. GE tubes have relatively poor durability and high reintervention rates compared with other endoscopic techniques. A single-center retrospective care series on 102 pediatric patients over a 9-year period demonstrated variable, but high rates of tube replacements (mean, 2.2; range, 1–14) over a median duration of 39 days (range, 2–474 days).[65] Further, in patients without significant anorexia, the inability to eat by mouth can have significant implications on health-related quality of life, a phenomenon that can be extrapolated from data in patients with esophageal cancer.[66]

Enteral Stents

For decades, the mainstay of the endoscopic therapy of malignant GOO has been endoscopically placed enteral stents. The design and materials of the stents have evolved over time, and currently most manufactures are producing uncovered metal stents made of nickel and titanium alloys, most commonly nitinol.[67] The technique involves advancing a guidewire beyond the obstruction and opacifying the small bowel distal to the obstruction under fluoroscopic guidance (**Fig. 4**A, B). Once the length of the stricture is measured and the appropriate size stent selected, the stent is advanced on a compressed delivery system over the wire (**Fig. 4**C) and then deployed under fluoroscopic guidance (**Fig. 4**D). After deployment, stents will expand radially over time and the immediate waist seen after deployment (see **Fig. 4**D) will abate (**Fig. 4**E).

Compared with surgical bypass, enteral stents are associated with a quicker onset of symptom resolution, but higher rates of complications.[68] Hence these stents are preferable for patients with a shorter life expectancy (ie, ≤6 months), and this recommendation is supported by recently published guidelines from the American Society for Gastrointestinal Endoscopy.[68,69] Recurrence of GOO symptoms is frequently encountered with enteral stents as compared with surgical gastrojejunostomy, as shown in a small RCT, SUSTENT study.[68] A recent, large propensity score matched study[70] also confirmed superiority of surgical gastrojejunostomy in terms of patency and even survival. However, in clinical practice, patients often prefer less invasive endoscopic enteral stenting. In fact, in the SUSTENT study,[68] 38 of 77 eligible patients refused to the study enrollment because they preferred enteral stenting. Because the prognosis for advanced pancreatic cancer remains poor and the performance status of patients with GOO is often compromised, surgical gastrojejunostomy is performed

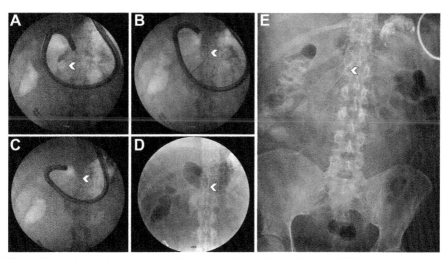

Fig. 4. The endoscopic placement of an enteral stent for malignant GOO from a tumor in the head of the pancreas. (*A*) After a wire (*arrowhead*) is passed beyond the obstruction, the downstream duodenum is opacified with a biliary extraction balloon (*arrowhead*) to delineate the length of the stricture. (*B*) The stent is advanced over the wire on a compressed delivery system (*arrowhead*). (*C*) The stent is deployed and (*D*) a significant waist is seen after endoscope removal (*arrowhead*). (*E*) This waist demonstrates near-complete abatement 2 days later on abdominal radiograph (*arrowhead*).

only in selected patients with good performance status, limited tumor burden, and longer life expectancy. For patients with resectable disease on neoadjuvant therapy, an enteral stent may be considered as a means to avoid a surgical bypass before a planned pancreaticoduodenectomy. Enteral stents that remain in place longer than 2 to 3 months duration are prone to failure, typically from obstruction owing to tissue ingrowth. In these instances, the most common reintervention is the placement of a second indwelling stent (either uncovered or partially covered), but recurrent failures are common. In the era of longer of neoadjuvant therapy, as well as the improved survival of patients undergoing palliative therapy, this limitation of enteral stent patency may one day result in its unseating as the first-line therapy for malignant GOO.

Enteral stents that cross the major papilla result in limitations and greater difficulty achieving subsequent biliary decompression, if needed. When placing enteral stents for malignant GOO in patients with native foregut anatomy, the need for concomitant or future biliary drainage is an important consideration to make. For obstructions occurring proximal to the level of the major papilla, care should be taken to choose the shortest possible stent to achieve palliation of the stricture and to place the stent in the most proximal location possible. Doing so will facilitate the ability to perform ERCP through the enteral stent, should the need arise. In circumstances when a previously placed enteral stent must cross the major papilla, ERCP can still be performed through the interstices of the enteral stent,[50,71–73] but clinical success rates are lower than conventional ERCP and, often, rendezvous techniques with interventional radiologists are required for retrograde biliary cannulation and stent placement (**Fig. 5**).[72] Outside of clinical centers with expertise in these endoscopic techniques, the placement of a percutaneous internal–external biliary drain is the most common modality of biliary decompression for patients with enteral stents obstructing the major papilla.

Endoscopic Ultrasound-Guided Gastroenterostomy

EUS-GE represents a newer technique whereby a de novo bypass tract is created with the use of a lumen-apposing metal stent. The first reported US experience with this technique was published in 2015, describing a 90% clinical success rate with no adverse events in 10 patients.[74] Recently, the procedure has become more refined, and several techniques to perform EUS-GE have been described.[75] A recent systematic review of 285 published cases describes a pooled technical success rate of 92%, a clinical success rate of 90%, an adverse event rate of 12%, and a reintervention rate of 9%.[76] Although most adverse events were minor, rare cases of gastric perforation and peritonitis requiring surgery, were reported.[76] Although the data surrounding this technique remain limited to retrospective cases series, a recent single-center cohort study retrospectively compared patients with malignant GOO undergoing enteral stent placement and EUS-GE. The study analyzed 78 consecutive patients with enteral stents and 22 consecutive patients with EUS-GE. The rate of stent failure was significantly higher in the enteral stent group (32.0% vs 8.3%; $P = .021$), and although the mean time to reintervention was similar between the enteral stent and EUS-GE groups (166 days vs 157 days; $P = .812$), a Kaplan–Meier survival analysis of time to repeat intervention significantly favored EUS-GE.[77] The impact, if any, of EUS-GE on the performance of subsequent pancreaticoduodenectomy remains unstudied to date.

Malignant Afferent Limb Syndrome

The complete or partial obstruction of the afferent (pancreaticobiliary) limb after pancreaticoduodenectomy most commonly occurs owing to radiation enteropathy or disease recurrence.[78,79] If this obstruction occurs downstream of the choledochojejunostomy or hepaticojejunostomy and pancreaticojejunostomy, this

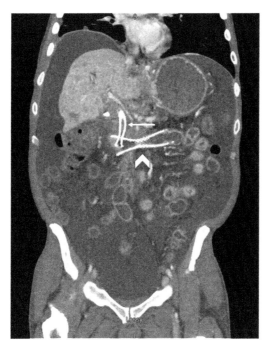

Fig. 5. Coronal CT images demonstrate a metal biliary stent (*arrow*) that was placed through a previously placed enteral stent (*arrowhead*).

results in afferent limb syndrome. The most common signs and symptoms of patients presenting with afferent limb syndrome include abdominal pain, nonproductive vomiting, jaundice, and cholangitis. In a large single-center series, the incidence of afferent limb syndrome after pancreaticoduodenectomy was reported to be 13%, occurring at a median of 1.2 years postoperatively.[79] Historically, afferent limb syndrome was treated with surgical bypass or percutaneous transhepatic biliary drains,[80–82] but endoscopic therapy has emerged as an efficacious first-line intervention for these patients.

The 2 main endoscopic therapies for afferent limb syndrome are enteral stents and EUS-GE. A case series and systematic review published in 2015 analyzed 52 patients with afferent limb syndrome, the majority of which were related to tumor recurrence. The patients were treated with either an endoscopic (40.0%), percutaneous (32.7%), surgical (11.5%), or conservative (15.4%) approaches.[78] The placement of enteral stents was technically successful in 87.5%.[78] The ability to place an enteral stent in patients with afferent limb syndrome depends on technical factors, such as the ability to reach the level of obstruction with the endoscope.

EUS-GE with lumen-apposing metal stents is emerging as the preferred endoscopic management technique for afferent limb syndrome.[83–92] The endosonographic target of EUS-GE in patients with afferent limb syndrome is typically a distended afferent limb that closely opposes the gastric wall (**Fig. 6**). PTBD, if present, can aid in further distention of the obstructed afferent limb and opacify it under fluoroscopy for targeting (see **Fig. 6**B).[83] A major advantage of this technique over an internal/external percutaneous drain is that it maintains the physiologic internal drainage of bile and pancreatic juice. Further, the placement of a large caliber lumen-apposing metal stents from the stomach into the afferent limb can facilitate endoscopic tissue acquisition if biopsy-proven tumor

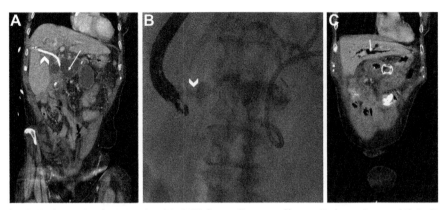

Fig. 6. Endoscopic ultrasound-guided GE for malignant afferent limb syndrome. (*A*) A distended, fluid-filled, afferent loop is seen (*arrow*). The patient has an internal/external biliary drain to temporize decompression (*arrowhead*). (*B*) The lumen-apposing metal stent is deployed and previously instilled contrast into the obstructed afferent limb immediately drains into the stomach (*arrowhead*). (*C*) This led to complete decompression of the afferent limb with pneumobilia (*arrow*).

recurrence would result in a change in therapy. Although there is reason for optimism based on early experience, more data are needed comparing EUS-GE to other techniques in managing afferent limb syndrome.

SUMMARY

In the management of pancreatic cancer, it is mandatory to get high-quality pancreas protocol imaging studies before performing invasive procedures such as EUS-FNA/FNB and ERCP. EUS-FFA/FNB plays a central role for tissue acquisition. The role of ERCP is limited in the diagnosis of pancreatic cancer but metal biliary stent placement via ERCP is the mainstay for palliation of MBO owing to pancreatic cancer. These stents can also be placed in those with resectable/borderline resectable pancreatic cancer where surgery is going to be delayed such as those receiving neoadjuvant therapy. Endoscopic enteral stenting is often selected for palliation of malignant GOO because of being less invasive but long-term patency is less compared with surgical gastrojejunostomy. Recently, EUS-guided interventions are increasingly being used as options for MBO and GOO. EUS-BD is now established as a rescue procedure after failed ERCP. EUS-gastrojejunostomy using a lumen-apposing metal stent can be a treatment option for GOO in the future.

CLINICS CARE POINTS

- High-quality pancreas protocol scan should be done before any invasive procedures such as EUS-FNA/FNB or ERCP.
- EUS with FNA/FNB is the preferred approach for tissue acquisition.
- Short expandable metal biliary stents can be placed safely for durable biliary drainage even in those with resectable pancreas cancer during neoadjuvant therapy.
- Endoscopic enteral stenting or EUS guided gastrojejunostomy can be an option in patients with gastric outlet obstruction.

DISCLOSURE

Y. Nakai: Nothing to disclose. Z. Smith: Nothing to disclose. K. J. Chang: Consulting with: Cook, Olympus, and Medtronic. K. S. Dua: Consulting with Boston Scientific.

REFERENCES

1. Siegel RL, Miller KD, Jemal A. Cancer statistics, 2020. CA Cancer J Clin 2020; 70(1):7–30.
2. Han J, Chang KJ. Endoscopic ultrasound-guided direct intervention for solid pancreatic tumors. Clin Endosc 2017;50(2):126–37.
3. Kitano M, Yoshida T, Itonaga M, et al. Impact of endoscopic ultrasonography on diagnosis of pancreatic cancer. J Gastroenterol 2019;54(1):19–32.
4. Krishna SG, Rao BB, Ugbarugba E, et al. Diagnostic performance of endoscopic ultrasound for detection of pancreatic malignancy following an indeterminate multidetector CT scan: a systemic review and meta-analysis. Surg Endosc 2017;31(11):4558–67.
5. Yang R, Lu M, Qian X, et al. Diagnostic accuracy of EUS and CT of vascular invasion in pancreatic cancer: a systematic review. J Cancer Res Clin Oncol 2014; 140(12):2077–86.
6. National Comprehensive Cancer Network. National Comprehensive Cancer Network (Version 1. 2020). Available at: https://www.nccn.org/professionals/physician_gls/pdf/pancreatic.pdf. Accessed December 2, 2020.
7. Unno M, Motoi F, Matsuyama Y, et al. Randomized phase II/III trial of neoadjuvant chemotherapy with gemcitabine and S-1 versus upfront surgery for resectable pancreatic cancer (Prep-02/JSAP-05). J Clin Oncol 2019;37(4_suppl):189.
8. Kurita A, Kodama Y, Nakamoto Y, et al. Impact of EUS-FNA for preoperative para-aortic lymph node staging in patients with pancreatobiliary cancer. Gastrointest Endosc 2016;84(3):467–75.e1.
9. Prasad P, Schmulewitz N, Patel A, et al. Detection of occult liver metastases during EUS for staging of malignancies. Gastrointest Endosc 2004;59(1):49–53.
10. Minaga K, Kitano M, Nakai A, et al. Improved detection of liver metastasis using Kupffer-phase imaging in contrast-enhanced harmonic EUS in patients with pancreatic cancer (with video). Gastrointest Endosc 2021;93(2):433–41.
11. Alberghina N, Sánchez-Montes C, Tuñón C, et al. Endoscopic ultrasonography can avoid unnecessary laparotomies in patients with pancreatic adenocarcinoma and undetected peritoneal carcinomatosis. Pancreatology 2017;17(5):858–64.
12. Vilmann P, Jacobsen GK, Henriksen FW, et al. Endoscopic ultrasonography with guided fine needle aspiration biopsy in pancreatic disease. Gastrointest Endosc 1992;38(2):172–3.
13. Chang KJ, Albers CG, Erickson RA, et al. Endoscopic ultrasound-guided fine needle aspiration of pancreatic carcinoma. Am J Gastroenterol 1994;89(2): 263–6.
14. Wang KX, Ben QW, Jin ZD, et al. Assessment of morbidity and mortality associated with EUS-guided FNA: a systematic review. Gastrointest Endosc 2011;73(2): 283–90.
15. Iglesias-Garcia J, Poley JW, Larghi A, et al. Feasibility and yield of a new EUS histology needle: results from a multicenter, pooled, cohort study. Gastrointest Endosc 2011;73(6):1189–96.
16. Iwashita T, Nakai Y, Samarasena JB, et al. High single-pass diagnostic yield of a new 25-gauge core biopsy needle for EUS-guided FNA biopsy in solid pancreatic lesions. Gastrointest Endosc 2013;77(6):909–15.

17. van Riet PA, Larghi A, Attili F, et al. A multicenter randomized trial comparing a 25-gauge EUS fine-needle aspiration device with a 20-gauge EUS fine-needle biopsy device. Gastrointest Endosc 2019;89(2):329–39.
18. Bang JY, Hebert-Magee S, Hasan MK, et al. Endoscopic ultrasonography-guided biopsy using a Franseen needle design: Initial assessment. Dig Endosc 2017; 29(3):338–46.
19. Bang JY, Hebert-Magee S, Navaneethan U, et al. Randomized trial comparing the Franseen and Fork-tip needles for EUS-guided fine-needle biopsy sampling of solid pancreatic mass lesions. Gastrointest Endosc 2018;87(6):1432–8.
20. Facciorusso A, Wani S, Triantafyllou K, et al. Comparative accuracy of needle sizes and designs for EUS tissue sampling of solid pancreatic masses: a network meta-analysis. Gastrointest Endosc 2019;90(6):893–903.e7.
21. Khan MA, Grimm IS, Ali B, et al. A meta-analysis of endoscopic ultrasound-fine-needle aspiration compared to endoscopic ultrasound-fine-needle biopsy: diagnostic yield and the value of onsite cytopathological assessment. Endosc Int Open 2017;5(5):E363–75.
22. Kandel P, Nassar A, Gomez V, et al. Comparison of endoscopic ultrasound-guided fine-needle biopsy versus fine-needle aspiration for genomic profiling and DNA yield in pancreatic cancer: a randomized crossover trial. Endoscopy 2021;53(4):376–82.
23. Hatfield AR, Smithies A, Wilkins R, et al. Assessment of endoscopic retrograde cholangio-pancreatography (ERCP) and pure pancreatic juice cytology in patients with pancreatic disease. Gut 1976;17(1):14–21.
24. Hanada K, Okazaki A, Hirano N, et al. Diagnostic strategies for early pancreatic cancer. J Gastroenterol 2015;50(2):147–54.
25. Kanno A, Masamune A, Hanada K, et al. Multicenter study of early pancreatic cancer in Japan. Pancreatology 2018;18(1):61–7.
26. Haba S, Yamao K, Bhatia V, et al. Diagnostic ability and factors affecting accuracy of endoscopic ultrasound-guided fine needle aspiration for pancreatic solid lesions: Japanese large single center experience. J Gastroenterol 2013;48(8): 973–81.
27. Ngamruengphong S, Swanson KM, Shah ND, et al. Preoperative endoscopic ultrasound-guided fine needle aspiration does not impair survival of patients with resected pancreatic cancer. Gut 2015;64(7):1105–10.
28. Yane K, Kuwatani M, Yoshida M, et al. Non-negligible rate of needle tract seeding after endoscopic ultrasound-guided fine-needle aspiration for patients undergoing distal pancreatectomy for pancreatic cancer. Dig Endosc 2020;32(5):801–11.
29. Speer AG, Cotton PB, Russell RC, et al. Randomised trial of endoscopic versus percutaneous stent insertion in malignant obstructive jaundice. Lancet 1987; 2(8550):57–62.
30. Smith AC, Dowsett JF, Russell RC, et al. Randomised trial of endoscopic stenting versus surgical bypass in malignant low bileduct obstruction. Lancet 1994; 344(8938):1655–60.
31. Davids PH, Groen AK, Rauws EA, et al. Randomised trial of self-expanding metal stents versus polyethylene stents for distal malignant biliary obstruction. Lancet 1992;340(8834-8835):1488–92.
32. Isayama H, Komatsu Y, Tsujino T, et al. A prospective randomised study of "covered" versus "uncovered" diamond stents for the management of distal malignant biliary obstruction. Gut 2004;53(5):729–34.
33. Kitano M, Yamashita Y, Tanaka K, et al. Covered self-expandable metal stents with an anti-migration system improve patency duration without increased

complications compared with uncovered stents for distal biliary obstruction caused by pancreatic carcinoma: a randomized multicenter trial. Am J Gastroenterol 2013;108(11):1713–22.

34. Tringali A, Hassan C, Rota M, et al. Covered vs. uncovered self-expandable metal stents for malignant distal biliary strictures: a systematic review and meta-analysis. Endoscopy 2018;50(6):631–41.

35. van der Gaag NA, Rauws EA, van Eijck CH, et al. Preoperative biliary drainage for cancer of the head of the pancreas. N Engl J Med 2010;362(2):129–37.

36. Tsujino T, Isayama H, Koike K. Preoperative drainage in pancreatic cancer. N Engl J Med 2010;362(14):1343–4 [author reply: 1346].

37. Tol JA, van Hooft JE, Timmer R, et al. Metal or plastic stents for preoperative biliary drainage in resectable pancreatic cancer. Gut 2016;65(12):1981–7.

38. Mullen JT, Lee JH, Gomez HF, et al. Pancreaticoduodenectomy after placement of endobiliary metal stents. J Gastrointest Surg 2005;9(8):1094–104 [discussion: 1104-5].

39. Wasan SM, Ross WA, Staerkel GA, et al. Use of expandable metallic biliary stents in resectable pancreatic cancer. Am J Gastroenterol 2005;100(9):2056–61.

40. Singal AK, Ross WA, Guturu P, et al. Self-expanding metal stents for biliary drainage in patients with resectable pancreatic cancer: single-center experience with 79 cases. Dig Dis Sci 2011;56(12):3678–84.

41. Aadam AA, Evans DB, Khan A, et al. Efficacy and safety of self-expandable metal stents for biliary decompression in patients receiving neoadjuvant therapy for pancreatic cancer: a prospective study. Gastrointest Endosc 2012;76(1):67–75.

42. Ballard DD, Rahman S, Ginnebaugh B, et al. Safety and efficacy of self-expanding metal stents for biliary drainage in patients receiving neoadjuvant therapy for pancreatic cancer. Endosc Int Open 2018;6(6):E714–21.

43. Boulay BR, Gardner TB, Gordon SR. Occlusion rate and complications of plastic biliary stent placement in patients undergoing neoadjuvant chemoradiotherapy for pancreatic cancer with malignant biliary obstruction. J Clin Gastroenterol 2010;44(6):452–5.

44. Seo DW, Sherman S, Dua KS, et al. Covered and uncovered biliary metal stents provide similar relief of biliary obstruction during neoadjuvant therapy in pancreatic cancer: a randomized trial. Gastrointest Endosc 2019;90(4):602–12.e4.

45. Giovannini M, Moutardier V, Pesenti C, et al. Endoscopic ultrasound-guided bilioduodenal anastomosis: a new technique for biliary drainage. Endoscopy 2001;33(10):898–900.

46. Sharaiha RZ, Khan MA, Kamal F, et al. Efficacy and safety of EUS-guided biliary drainage in comparison with percutaneous biliary drainage when ERCP fails: a systematic review and meta-analysis. Gastrointest Endosc 2017;85(5):904–14.

47. Nakai Y, Hamada T, Isayama H, et al. Endoscopic management of combined malignant biliary and gastric outlet obstruction. Dig Endosc 2017;29(1):16–25.

48. Hamada T, Isayama H, Nakai Y, et al. Duodenal invasion is a risk factor for the early dysfunction of biliary metal stents in unresectable pancreatic cancer. Gastrointest Endosc 2011;74(3):548–55.

49. Hamada T, Nakai Y, Isayama H, et al. Duodenal metal stent placement is a risk factor for biliary metal stent dysfunction: an analysis using a time-dependent covariate. Surg Endosc 2013;27(4):1243–8.

50. Khashab MA, Valeshabad AK, Leung W, et al. Multicenter experience with performance of ERCP in patients with an indwelling duodenal stent. Endoscopy 2014;46(3):252–5.

51. Hamada T, Isayama H, Nakai Y, et al. Transmural biliary drainage can be an alternative to transpapillary drainage in patients with an indwelling duodenal stent. Dig Dis Sci 2014;59(8):1931–8.

52. Nakai Y, Sato T, Hakuta R, et al. Long-term outcomes of a long, partially covered metal stent for EUS-guided hepaticogastrostomy in patients with malignant biliary obstruction (with video). Gastrointest Endosc 2020;92(3):623–31.e1.

53. Ogura T, Chiba Y, Masuda D, et al. Comparison of the clinical impact of endoscopic ultrasound-guided choledochoduodenostomy and hepaticogastrostomy for bile duct obstruction with duodenal obstruction. Endoscopy 2016;48(2): 156–63.

54. Bang JY, Navaneethan U, Hasan M, et al. Stent placement by EUS or ERCP for primary biliary decompression in pancreatic cancer: a randomized trial (with videos). Gastrointest Endosc 2018;88(1):9–17.

55. Paik WH, Lee TH, Park DH, et al. EUS-guided biliary drainage versus ERCP for the primary palliation of malignant biliary obstruction: a multicenter randomized clinical trial. Am J Gastroenterol 2018;113(7):987–97.

56. Park JK, Woo YS, Noh DH, et al. Efficacy of EUS-guided and ERCP-guided biliary drainage for malignant biliary obstruction: prospective randomized controlled study. Gastrointest Endosc 2018;88(2):277–82.

57. Tsuchiya T, Teoh AYB, Itoi T, et al. Long-term outcomes of EUS-guided choledochoduodenostomy using a lumen-apposing metal stent for malignant distal biliary obstruction: a prospective multicenter study. Gastrointest Endosc 2018;87(4): 1138–46.

58. Wong YT, Brams DM, Munson L, et al. Gastric outlet obstruction secondary to pancreatic cancer: surgical vs endoscopic palliation. Surg Endosc 2002;16(2): 310–2.

59. Jang S, Stevens T, Lopez R, et al. Superiority of gastrojejunostomy over endoscopic stenting for palliation of malignant gastric outlet obstruction. Clin Gastroenterol Hepatol 2019;17(7):1295–302.e1.

60. Jang SH, Lee H, Min BH, et al. Palliative gastrojejunostomy versus endoscopic stent placement for gastric outlet obstruction in patients with unresectable gastric cancer: a propensity score-matched analysis. Surg Endosc 2017;31(10): 4217–23.

61. Upchurch E, Ragusa M, Cirocchi R. Stent placement versus surgical palliation for adults with malignant gastric outlet obstruction. Cochrane Database Syst Rev 2018;5:CD012506.

62. Byrne KR, Fang JC. Endoscopic placement of enteral feeding catheters. Curr Opin Gastroenterol 2006;22(5):546–50.

63. Lang GD, Mullady DK, Kushnir VM. A novel through-the-snare technique for percutaneous endoscopic gastrojejunostomy tube placement. VideoGIE 2017; 2(9):225–6.

64. Sibille A, Glorieux D, Fauville JP, et al. An easier method for percutaneous endoscopic gastrojejunostomy tube placement. Gastrointest Endosc 1998;48(5): 514–7.

65. Fortunato JE, Darbari A, Mitchell SE, et al. The limitations of gastro-jejunal (G-J) feeding tubes in children: a 9-year pediatric hospital database analysis. Am J Gastroenterol 2005;100(1):186–9.

66. Smith ZL, Gonzaga JE, Haasler GB, et al. Self-expanding metal stents improve swallowing and maintain nutrition during neoadjuvant therapy for esophageal cancer. Dig Dis Sci 2017;62(6):1647–56.

67. Committee AT, Varadarajulu S, Banerjee S, et al. Enteral stents. Gastrointest Endosc 2011;74(3):455–64.
68. Jeurnink SM, Steyerberg EW, van Hooft JE, et al. Surgical gastrojejunostomy or endoscopic stent placement for the palliation of malignant gastric outlet obstruction (SUSTENT study): a multicenter randomized trial. Gastrointest Endosc 2010; 71(3):490–9.
69. Committee ASoP, Jue TL, Storm AC, et al. ASGE guideline on the role of endoscopy in the management of benign and malignant gastroduodenal obstruction. Gastrointest Endosc 2021;93(2):309–22.e4.
70. Jang S, Stevens T, Lopez R, et al. Superiority of gastrojejunostomy over endoscopic stenting for palliation of malignant gastric outlet obstruction. Clin Gastroenterol Hepatol 2019;17(7):1295–302.e1.
71. Staub J, Siddiqui A, Taylor LJ, et al. ERCP performed through previously placed duodenal stents: a multicenter retrospective study of outcomes and adverse events. Gastrointest Endosc 2018;87(6):1499–504.
72. Lee JJ, Hyun JJ, Choe JW, et al. Endoscopic biliary stent insertion through specialized duodenal stent for combined malignant biliary and duodenal obstruction facilitated by stent or PTBD guidance. Scand J Gastroenterol 2017; 52(11):1258–62.
73. Vanbiervliet G, Demarquay JF, Dumas R, et al. Endoscopic insertion of biliary stents in 18 patients with metallic duodenal stents who developed secondary malignant obstructive jaundice. Gastroenterol Clin Biol 2004;28(12):1209–13.
74. Khashab MA, Kumbhari V, Grimm IS, et al. EUS-guided gastroenterostomy: the first U.S. clinical experience (with video). Gastrointest Endosc 2015;82(5):932–8.
75. Irani S, Itoi T, Baron TH, et al. EUS-guided gastroenterostomy: techniques from East to West. VideoGIE 2020;5(2):48–50.
76. Iqbal U, Khara HS, Hu Y, et al. EUS-guided gastroenterostomy for the management of gastric outlet obstruction: a systematic review and meta-analysis. Endosc Ultrasound 2020;9(1):16–23.
77. Ge PS, Young JY, Dong W, et al. EUS-guided gastroenterostomy versus enteral stent placement for palliation of malignant gastric outlet obstruction. Surg Endosc 2019;33(10):3404–11.
78. Huang J, Hao S, Yang F, et al. Endoscopic metal enteral stent placement for malignant afferent loop syndrome after pancreaticoduodenectomy. Wideochir Inne Tech Maloinwazyjne 2015;10(2):257–65.
79. Pannala R, Brandabur JJ, Gan SI, et al. Afferent limb syndrome and delayed GI problems after pancreaticoduodenectomy for pancreatic cancer: single-center, 14-year experience. Gastrointest Endosc 2011;74(2):295–302.
80. Aimoto T, Uchida E, Nakamura Y, et al. Malignant afferent loop obstruction following pancreaticoduodenectomy: report of two cases. J Nippon Med Sch 2006;73(4):226–30.
81. Caldicott DG, Ziprin P, Morgan R. Transhepatic insertion of a metallic stent for the relief of malignant afferent loop obstruction. Cardiovasc Intervent Radiol 2000; 23(2):138–40.
82. Chevallier P, Novellas S, Motamedi JP, et al. Percutaneous jejunostomy and stent placement for treatment of malignant Roux-en-Y obstruction: a case report. Clin Imaging 2006;30(4):283–6.
83. Adoor D, Smith ZL. Percutaneous- and EUS-guided gastroenterostomy for malignant afferent limb syndrome. VideoGIE 2020;5(11):542–4.
84. El Bacha H, Leblanc S, Bordacahar B, et al. Endoscopic ultrasound-guided enteroenterostomy for afferent limb syndrome. ACG Case Rep J 2020;7(8):e00442.

85. Ghoz H, Foulks C, Gomez V. Management of afferent limb obstruction by use of EUS-guided creation of a jejunojejunostomy and placement of a lumen-apposing metal stent. VideoGIE 2019;4(7):337–40.

86. Irani S. Placing a lumen-apposing metal stent despite ascites: feasibility and safety. VideoGIE 2020;5(11):586–90.

87. Ligresti D, Amata M, Messina M, et al. Single-step EUS-guided jejunojejunostomy with a lumen-apposing metal stent as treatment for malignant afferent limb syndrome. VideoGIE 2020;5(4):154–6.

88. Shah A, Khanna L, Sethi A. Treatment of afferent limb syndrome: novel approach with endoscopic ultrasound-guided creation of a gastrojejunostomy fistula and placement of lumen-apposing stent. Endoscopy 2015;47(Suppl 1 UCTN): E309–10.

89. Hamada T, Hakuta R, Takahara N, et al. Covered versus uncovered metal stents for malignant gastric outlet obstruction: Systematic review and meta-analysis. Dig Endosc 2017;29(3):259–71.

90. Khashab MA, Bukhari M, Baron TH, et al. International multicenter comparative trial of endoscopic ultrasonography-guided gastroenterostomy versus surgical gastrojejunostomy for the treatment of malignant gastric outlet obstruction. Endosc Int Open 2017;5(4):E275–81.

91. Chen YI, Itoi T, Baron TH, et al. EUS-guided gastroenterostomy is comparable to enteral stenting with fewer re-interventions in malignant gastric outlet obstruction. Surg Endosc 2017;31(7):2946–52.

92. Itoi T, Baron TH, Khashab MA, et al. Technical review of endoscopic ultrasonography-guided gastroenterostomy in 2017. Dig Endosc 2017;29(4):495–502.

Current Controversies in Neoadjuvant Therapy for Pancreatic Cancer

Erin P. Ward, MD[a], Herbert J. Zeh III, MD[b], Susan Tsai, MD, MHS[a],*

KEYWORDS

- Pancreatic cancer • Neoadjuvant therapy • Micro-metastatic disease • CA19-9

KEY POINTS

- Despite universal recommendation for adjuvant therapy only 50% of patients will receive therapy. Treatment is determined by the patient's ability to recover from surgery.
- Neoadjuvant therapy allows for the early delivery of chemotherapy and assessment of response. Treatment is determined by the tumor response and tumor biology.
- Although the role of neoadjuvant therapy has gained acceptance, there is significant controversy regarding the type and duration of chemotherapy and the utility of neoadjuvant radiation.

INTRODUCTION

Almost three decades after the initial report of the use of preoperative (neoadjuvant) therapy for pancreatic ductal adenocarcinoma (PDAC), we have reached an inflection point in the acceptance and even embrace of neoadjuvant therapy as the preferred treatment sequencing for patients with operable PDAC.[1] The arc of progress has evolved from prioritization of surgical resection above all other therapies to an acknowledgment of the need for multimodality therapy.[2–6] Incremental advances in clinical medicine and rapid acceleration of scientific discoveries have transformed our understanding of PDAC biology and positioned us to make significant progress in the management of PDAC in the next decade. In this article, we will review the rationale for neoadjuvant therapy, focus on oncologic outcomes using neoadjuvant therapy, and discuss current controversies regarding neoadjuvant therapy sequencing in the treatment of PDAC.

[a] Surgical Oncology Division, Department of Surgery, Medical College of Wisconsin, 8701 W Watertown Plank Road, Milwaukee, WI 53226, USA; [b] Division of Surgical Oncology, Department of Surgery, UT Southwestern (University of Texas), 5323 Harry Hines Blvd. Dallas, TX 75390, USA
* Corresponding author.
E-mail address: stsai@mcw.edu

Surg Oncol Clin N Am 30 (2021) 657–671
https://doi.org/10.1016/j.soc.2021.06.010
1055-3207/21/© 2021 Elsevier Inc. All rights reserved.

surgonc.theclinics.com

Pitfalls of Adjuvant Treatment Sequencing

A diagnosis of PDAC induces a nihilism that is not encountered in many other diseases.[7] Underutilization of surgery even among patients with potentially operable PDAC continues to persist and is likely driven in part by the perception that disease recurrence occurs quickly after surgery.[7,8] Historically, patients with operable PDAC who did not receive any postoperative (adjuvant) therapy experienced a median progression free survival of only 7 months.[6] Indeed, after the landmark CONKO-001 clinical trial, adjuvant therapy became the standard for all patients with resected PDAC, regardless of stage.[6] Over the past two decades, there has been an evolving understanding of PDAC as being a systemic disease, with evidence that circulating tumor cells can be detected, in animal models, even before an pancreatic tumor can be detected by imaging.[9,10] The addition of adjuvant therapy is a logical approach to the management of micrometastatic disease and has been effective in other solid organ tumors.[11,12] Indeed, the unequivocal benefit of postoperative (adjuvant) chemotherapy to improve overall and disease-free survival has been demonstrated for patients with operable PDAC by successive clinical trials as well.[6,13]

Adjuvant therapy, by definition, places the most difficult aspect of multimodality therapy (surgery) first, and any resultant complication from surgery can impede the subsequent delivery of other therapies. This is an important consideration when interpreting adjuvant trials which enroll patients after they have recovered from surgery. It is of particular significance with regard to pancreatic surgery, where 30% to 40% of patients experience complications.[14,15] As a result, 40% to 50% of postoperative patients will never recover to receive adjuvant therapy, and this is independent of whether if they received a surgery-first approach or a preoperative (neoadjuvant) therapy approach.[15,16] To account for the exclusion of this large proportion of, patients would need to be enrolled before or at the time of surgery. The impact of presurgical enrollment on the outcomes of a surgery-first treatment approach can be seen by comparing two recent PRODIGE-24 and ESPAC-5F trials. The PRODIGE 24-ACCORD adjuvant trial has garnered much attention for the superior survival outcomes experienced with adjuvant FOLFIRINOX. The trial compared adjuvant FOLFIRINOX to adjuvant gemcitabine chemotherapy and reported 3-year overall survival rates of 63% among patients who received adjuvant FOLFIRINOX as compared to 48% among patients in the gemcitabine control arm.[17] Although this was a multicentered international trial, on average only 1.4 patients were accrued per center each year, suggesting that these were a highly selected group of patients. In contrast, in the recent ESPAC-5F trial, which randomly assigned patients to surgery-first or neoadjuvant therapy and in the surgery-first arm, patients with PDAC who were enrolled before surgery. Among those patients who were assigned to the immediate surgery arm, only 62% of patients underwent resection, and the 1-year overall survival rate for this arm was only 40%.[18] The inability to predictably deliver adjuvant systemic therapy to a large proportion of patients with PDAC is the most compelling argument against a surgery-first approach. As with other solid tumors, a neoadjuvant treatment approach has become the preferred approach to prioritize and effectively deliver systemic therapy to patients with high risk of micrometastatic disease.

Advantages of a Neoadjuvant Treatment Approach

Neoadjuvant therapy was originally conceived to identify patients at the highest risk to develop early postoperative metastatic disease. After up-front surgical resection, a staggering 77% of recurrences happen within a median of 12 months.[19] With a neoadjuvant approach, some of the patients who would have had an early recurrence are identified during the neoadjuvant treatment before surgery. Across several clinical trials, approximately 30% of patients with localized PDAC developed metastatic disease progression while receiving neoadjuvant therapy (**Table 1**).[20–22] The survival of this cohort of patients mirrors the survival of patients who present with metastatic disease; therefore, a neoadjuvant approach spares these patients the morbidity of an unnecessary surgery and obviates any surgically related delay in delivering additional therapy. The obvious benefit of identifying such patients is that they are spared unnecessary morbidity without any delay in the delivery of systemic therapy—an important consideration in this era of improved multiagent chemotherapy. For those patients who are able to complete neoadjuvant therapy and surgery, the delivery of neoadjuvant therapy has been associated with pathologic downstaging of the primary tumor. Rates of lymph node positive disease with up-front surgery have been reported between 73% and 80%, and margin positive (R1) resections range from 43% to 60%.[13,23] The addition of neoadjuvant therapy has been associated with lower rates of lymph node–positive disease (38%–50%) and R1 resections (10%–25%) (**Table 1**).[20,22,24,25] Importantly, nodal downstaging has been associated with improved overall survival.[26] In addition, neoadjuvant therapy is not associated with increased perioperative morbidity or mortality. An NSQIP study identified 1562 patients who received neoadjuvant therapy for pancreatic cancer.[27] There were no differences in 30-day mortality or postoperative morbidity between patients who received neoadjuvant therapy versus a surgery-first approach. Indeed, neoadjuvant chemoradiation was associated with decreased rates of pancreatic fistula.[27] The final advantage of a neoadjuvant approach is the ability to monitor treatment response. Unlike in the adjuvant setting, where there is no tumor remaining to assess treatment response, in the neoadjuvant setting, response to therapy can be monitored and treatment can be changed accordingly.

As the experience with neoadjuvant therapy for localized PDAC has matured, several meta-analyses of single institutional experiences have been performed to examine the outcomes of patients treated with neoadjuvant therapy. In a meta-analysis of 5520 patients who received neoadjuvant therapy for localized pancreatic cancer,[28] neoadjuvant therapy was associated with 0% mortality, 5% biliary complications, and 21% hospitalization rate. Margin negative resection rates exceeded 80% after neoadjuvant therapy, and the median overall survival after neoadjuvant therapy and surgery was 30 months and 27 months for patients with resectable and borderline resectable disease, respectively. The Dutch Pancreatic Cancer Group compared the outcomes of 3484 patients with resectable or borderline resectable PDAC who were treated with either a neoadjuvant or surgery-first approach.[29] Neoadjuvant therapy was associated with higher rates of node negative disease (65% vs 43%, $P < .001$) and higher rates of margin negative resection (87% vs 67%, $P < .001$). The median overall survival among patients who were treated with neoadjuvant therapy 26 months versus 15 months. Recently Cloyd and colleagues published a meta-analysis of randomized control studies including 850 patients with either borderline or resectable disease treated with gemcitabine based neoadjuvant therapy or up-front surgery (30). Overall neoadjuvant therapy was associated with improved overall survival (hazard ratio [HR] 0.73), similar rates of resection, and improved rates of R0 resections and negative nodal disease.

Several recent randomized clinical trials have compared a surgery-first approach for resectable and/or borderline resectable patients to a neoadjuvant approach (**Table 2**). The PREOPANC trial randomized 246 patients with resectable or borderline PDAC to preoperative gemcitabine-based chemoradiation followed by surgery and four cycles of adjuvant gemcitabine to up-front surgery followed by 6 cycles

Table 1
Neoadjuvant phase II trials for pancreatic cancer (resectable and borderline)

Author, Year	Trial Design	n	Treatment	Completion of Neoadjuvant Therapy and Surgery, n (%)	Resection Rate (N, %)	R0 Resection (%, N)	Node Positive Disease (N, %)	pCR (N, %)	Median OS of Resected Patients
Evans et al,[1] 1992	Single Institution	28, Resectable	50.4 Gy+ 5FU	28, 100%	17, 61%	14, 82%	5,29%	0	NR
Talamonti et al,[56] 2006	Phase II, multi-institutional	20, Resectable	36 Gy + gemcitabine	19, 95%	17, 85%	16, 94%	6, 35%	1, 5%	26 mo
Evans et al,[20] 2008	Phase II, single institution	86, Resectable	30 Gy + gemcitabine	86, 100%	64, 74%	58, 89%	24, 38%	1, 2%	34 mo
Heinrich et al,[57] 2008	Phase II, single institution	28, Resectable	Gemcitabine + cisplatin	18, 64%	25, 89%	20, 80%	19, 76%	0	19 mo
Kim et al,[58] 2013	Phase II Trial, multi-institutional	68, Resectable and Borderline	Gemcitabine + Oxaliplatin +30 Gy	66, 97%	43, 63%	36, 84%	36, 84%	NR	27.1 mo
Katz et al,[59] 2016	Phase II, multi-institutional	22, Borderline	FOLFIRINOX + 50 Gy chemoradiation with capecitabine	21, 95%	15, 68%	14, 93%	5, 33%	2, 13%	~22 mo
Murphy et al,[60] 2018	Phase II, single institution	48, Borderline	FOLFIRINOX + 30 Gy or 50 Gy chemoradiation with capecitabine or 5FU	39, 81%	32, 82%	31, 97%	12, 38%	0	NR
Wei et al,[61] 2019	Phase II Trial, multi-institutional	114, Resectable	Gemcitabine + erlotinib	114, 100%	83, 73%	67,81%	59, 71%	NR	25.4 mo

Abbreviations: Gy, Gray; pCR, pathologic complete response; R0, negative margins.

Table 2
Randomized controlled trials for resectable pancreatic cancer comparing neoadjuvant chemotherapy with up-front surgery

Study	Trial Design	Number of Patients, Resectability	Neoadjuvant Therapy (NT) Compared to Up-Front Surgery (UFS)	Adjuvant Therapy	Resection Rate (%)		R0 Rate (%)		N0 Rate (%)		Overall Survival (mo)		HR of NT (95% CI)
					NT	UFS	NT	UFS	NT	UFS	NT	UFS	
Neoadjuvant Chemotherapy vs. UFS													
Unno et al,[62] 2019	Phase II/III, multi-institution	362, Resectable	Gemcitabine and S1	S1	76.9	72.2	N/A	N/A	N/A	N/A	36.7	26.6	0.72 [0.55–0.94]
Versteijne et al,[30] 2020	Phase III, multi-institution	246, Resectable/ borderline resectable	Perioperative chemoradiation	Gemcitabine	61	72	71	40	67	22	16.0	14.3	0.73 [0.56–0.96]

Abbreviations: HR, hazard ratio; N0, node negative; NT, neoadjuvant therapy; R0, negative margins; UFS, up-front surgery.

of adjuvant gemcitabine. Neoadjuvant therapy was associated with improved R0 resection rates (71% vs 40%), lower rates of positive lymph nodes, and improved DFS.[24] Updated 3- and 5-year overall survival by intention-to-treat analysis was presented at the 2021 meeting of the American Society of Clinical Oncology. There was an improvement in overall survival at both 3 years (27.7% vs 16.5%) and 5 years (20.5% vs 6.5%, $P = .025$).[30] The ESPAC-5F trial randomized patients with borderline resectable disease to either neoadjuvant gemcitabine/capecitabine, FOLFIRINOX, capecitabine-based chemoradiation, or surgery-first.[18] All resected patients received adjuvant therapy. Overall, no significant difference in resection rates were observed between the neoadjuvant arms and the surgery-first arm. The 1-year survival rate was 40% for patients who underwent up-front surgical resection compared with 77% for patients who received neoadjuvant therapy ($P < .001$). These randomized trials have further cemented the role of neoadjuvant therapy for patients with operable pancreatic cancer.

Currently, consensus guidelines recommend neoadjuvant therapy for patients with borderline resectable and locally advanced PDAC, as anatomically they are at the highest possible risk for a margin positive resection.[31] The management of patients with resectable PDAC is more controversial, although many may argue that the challenges of delivery adjuvant therapy are immutable regardless of stage. Nevertheless, several ongoing trials comparing surgery-first versus neoadjuvant therapy are actively accruing or have pending results are summarized in **Table 3**. The ALLIANCE 021806 trial (NCT04340141), which randomizes up-front surgical resection and adjuvant therapy with perioperative chemotherapy, will seek to definitively address the value of neoadjuvant therapy in patients with resectable disease.

Pitfalls of Neoadjuvant Therapy

Although there is a growing consensus to use neoadjuvant therapy as the preferred treatment sequence for patients with operable PDAC, the implementation can be challenging and requires the engagement of a multidisciplinary team to effectively manage potential complications. In addition, a neoadjuvant approach is incumbent on establishing a tissue diagnosis before treatment and the need for durable biliary decompression.

Histologic tissue confirmation is generally required before the initiation of chemotherapy or radiation. Obtaining tissue can be a challenge depending on the local endoscopic capabilities and the location of the tumor. Although several studies have shown overall high overall accuracy, some patients may require multiple attempts to get adequate tissue diagnosis.[32,33] Infrequently, it can take more than one sample to obtain appropriate tissue for diagnosis and has the potential to delay therapy initiation. Although relatively rare, up to 6% of patients can have complications related to the biopsy, although these are most commonly self-limited.[33]

Resolution of biliary obstruction is also required to deliver many chemotherapies. In general, self-expanding metal stents have been the preferred method of biliary drainage in patients who receive neoadjuvant therapy, as the patency rates are significantly better than those of silastic/polyethylene stents.[34] Complications associated with metal stents include stent occlusion, migration, and kinking, all of which can contribute to the development of cholecystitis or cholangitis.[35,36] Fortunately, stent-associated complications are relatively infrequent and most can be managed nonoperatively. Approximately 1% to 4% of patients may require reintervention to maintain stent patency and with up to 15% of patients can have stent cholangitis requiring antibiotics, admissions, and/or stent exchange.[37] Other complications include stent-associated acute cholecystitis among patients with localized or metastatic

Table 3
Pending neoadjuvant trials for pancreatic cancer

Study, Study Design. (NCT#)	Treatment Arms	Primary Endpoints	Secondary Endpoints	Anticipated Accrual Period
Alliance A021806, Phase III Randomized Trial (NCT 04340141)	1. mFOLFIRINOX (8 cycles) followed by surgery and 4 cycles of adjuvant mFOLFIRINOX 2. Surgery followed by 12 cycles of mFOLFIRINOX	Overall Survival	Disease free survival, time to locoregional recurrence, time to distant metastases, R0 resection rate, rate of resectability, pathologic complete response	July 2020 - November 2030
Nordic Pancreatic Cancer Trial (NorPact-1), Phase III Randomized Trial (NCT 02919787)	1. mFOLFIRINOX (4 cycles), Surgery, then 4 cycles of Gemcitabine 2. Surgery followed by 6 cycles of Gemcitabine	Overall Survival at 18 mo after randomization	Mortality at 1 y after treatment starts, disease free survival, histopathologic response, complication rate after surgery	September 2016, October 2021
Neoadjuvant Treatment in Resectable Pancreatic Cancer, Phase III Randomized Trial (NEOPA) (NCT 01900327)	1. Neoadjuvant 50 Gy chemoradiation with Gemcitabine for 6 cycles, Surgery, then adjuvant chemotherapy (preferably 6 cycles Gemcitabine) 2. Surgery followed by 6 cycles of Gemcitabine	3-y Overall Survival	R0 resection, frequency of toxicity events, resectability rate, intraoperative irregularities, postoperative complications, disease progression during neoadjuvant therapy	February 2015, November 2016
Neo-adjuvant FOLF(IRIN)OX for Resectable Pancreatic Adenocarcinoma (PANACHE 01- PRODIGE 48) (NCT 02959879)	1. Neoadjuvant FOLFOX (4 cycles), Surgery, then 8 cycles of adjuvant chemotherapy 2. Neoadjuvant FOLFIRIONX (4 cycles), Surgery, then 8 cycles of adjuvant chemotherapy 3. Surgery, 12 cycles of standard chemotherapy	12 mo overall survival after surgery, completion of chemotherapy treatment sequence	Treatment-related adverse events, postoperative complication rates, R0 resection rate,	March 2017, December 2021

Abbreviations: R0, negative margins.

periampullary tumors ranges from 6% to 10%.[38–40] In general, acute cholecystitis during neoadjuvant treatment is best managed with a temporizing cholecystostomy tube to avoid interruption of neoadjuvant therapy.[41] A cholecystectomy can be performed later at the time of the pancreaticoduodenectomy.

The neoadjuvant therapy regimens are not without toxicity, and for some patients, the toxicity of the therapy limits their ability to stay on treatment and can require temporary breaks from treatment, admission or even cessation of treatment. Up to 64% of patients may experience some kind of toxicity associated with treatment, most commonly gastrointestinal or hematological in nature.[29] Although the attrition rates in the neoadjuvant setting are significantly better than those in the adjuvant studies, toxicities can lead to a delay in surgery. The toxicity related to neoadjuvant therapy has also been cited as a potential risk for increased risks of morbidity and mortality after surgery, although this has not been observed in the large retrospective or meta-analysis studies.[42] Overall the rates of complications postoperatively after neoadjuvant therapy versus up-front surgery are not significantly different.[27]

The most commonly cited concern regarding neoadjuvant therapy is that some patients may progress locally and lose their window for resection.[20,22] In reality, isolated local progression is very rare, and most patients who progress on therapy develop distant disease in the liver, peritoneum, or lungs.[25] These patients are often those with biologically aggressive disease or chemotherapy resistant disease that would ultimately have rapidly progressed after surgery. In contrast, several meta-analyses have demonstrated that neoadjuvant therapy is more commonly associated with downstaging of local disease, rather than progression.[29,43]

Current Controversies

Defining the optimal neoadjuvant therapy

Although there is a growing acceptance for neoadjuvant therapy for the management of localized PDAC, the type of therapy and duration of therapy remains controversial. At this time, the two common primary systemic therapies are gemcitabine-nab-paclitaxel or FOLFIRINOX. The SWOG S1505 trial randomized patients with resectable PDAC to 12 weeks of preoperative modified FOLFIRINOX or gemcitabine plus nab-paclitaxel followed by additional 12 weeks of adjuvant therapy.[42] The study failed to show superiority of either regimen in a pick-the-winner design to a prespecified endpoint of 2-year overall survival. In addition, median disease-free survival, R0 resection and completion of intended therapy rates were similar between both arms. Although common toxicities varied between the two arms, the rates of grade III and IV toxicities were similar. At this time, there is no clear superior regimen.

The unanswered question is whether there a way to predict which therapy a patient is more likely to respond. There have been great advancements in molecular subtyping of PDAC, and there are multiple proposed classifications for pancreas tumors. Some studies suggest that classical and basal subtype tumors (Moffit classification) may be predictive response to FOLFIRINOX.[44,45] The challenge with implementing molecular profiling of pancreatic tumors is obtaining adequate cellularity from endoscopic ultrasound guided biopsies. A recent phase II trial was completed documenting the feasibility of using molecular profiling based on endoscopic fine needle aspiration biopsies to select treatment based on mutations associated with gemcitabine resistance.[25] Overall 73% of patients had adequate cellularity to allow for the immunocytochemical profiling to select an agent. The median overalls survival of patients who completed all neoadjuvant therapy and surgery was 45 months.

Beyond FOLFIRNOX and gemcitabine-based systemic therapies, additional agents are being utilized in the metastatic setting among patients with germline mutations affecting the homologous directed repair pathway. Cancers arising in the setting of a BRCA mutation are associated with increased sensitivity to platinum due to ineffective DNA repair. The most prominent example is the use of olaparib in patients with metastatic PDAC with a BRCA 1 or 2 mutation. The POLO study demonstrated that patients with metastatic PDAC had significantly longer mOS if treated with maintenance olaparib versus placebo following a progression free interval on a first-line platinum-based chemotherapy.[46] Additional studies have looked at the benefits of using platinum agents in these patients. Recent phase II studies show that patients with stage III and IV PDAC in with a *BRCA* mutation or PALB2 mutation have good responses to gemcitabine and cisplatin. These studies are leading the way in precision medicine for PDAC, the robust responses seen in the locally advanced or metastatic setting may have future implications for neoadjuvant therapies.[47]

The optimal duration of neoadjuvant therapy for resectable versus borderline resectable PDAC also remains controversial. Currently neoadjuvant treatment is based on completing a prescribed number of cycles chemotherapy or a prescribed number of chemoradiation treatments. This is also true of adjuvant therapy. At this time, there is no clear consensus as to how much chemotherapy should be received before surgery and whether this should vary based on stage of disease (resectable versus borderline resectable).

In other solid organ tumors, there has been a move away from a perioperative "sandwich approach" treatment to a total neoadjuvant approach. The total neoadjuvant approach is also being utilized for borderline and locally advanced tumors both a clinical trial and general practice.[48,49] Total neoadjuvant regimens may provide additional benefits to a perioperative treatment regimen, as it may allow for more patients to complete the entire course of therapy by avoiding high attrition rates in the adjuvant setting and allow physicians the opportunity to switch treatments during a mid-treatment restaging.

Re-evaluating treatment response

Restaging and evaluation of treatment response, either in the middle of a total neoadjuvant setting or before surgery, can be challenging. Although CT scans are the cornerstone of response assessment, there is not always a significant change in appearance of local tumor that can be clearly defined as improved or worse. Additional adjuncts, such as carbohydrate 19-9 (CA19-9) monitoring can be used to supplement CT findings. A decrease in CA19-9 in response to neoadjuvant therapy has been shown to correlate with overall survival, and the normalization of CA19-9 has been a strong favorable prognostic marker.[50–52] In contrast, a rise in CA19-9 while on neoadjuvant therapy has been associated with metastatic disease in up to 50% of cases. At this time, there is no clear guidelines on how to incorporate biomarker response in the neoadjuvant setting, or how much of a change in CA19-9 qualifies as a significant response. In the era of high-quality CT scans, with the ability to monitor both the primary tumor response to therapy and tumor markers for CA19-9 producing tumors, one could argue that the timing of therapy should be goal-orientated and adaptive. Currently at least one clinical trial is accruing to evaluate if an adaptive approach to neoadjuvant therapy in response to radiographic and CA19-9 changes and patient performance status after 2 months of therapy can lead to improved patient outcomes (NCT 03322995).

Use of Radiation for Operable Pancreatic Cancer

The utility of neoadjuvant chemoradiation remains highly controversial. Although chemoradiation was used in many of the early neoadjuvant studies showing improved R0

Table 4
Randomized controlled trials for resectable or borderline resectable pancreatic cancer comparing chemoradiation with up-front surgery

Study	Trial Design	Number of Patients, Resectability	Neoadjuvant Therapy (NT) Compared With Up-Front Surgery (UFS)	Adjuvant Therapy	Resection Rate (%)		R0 Rate (%)		N0 Rate (%)		Overall Survival (mo)		HR of NT (95% CI)
					NT	UFS	NT	UFS	NT	UFS	NT	UFS	
Neoadjuvant chemoradiation vs UFS													
Golcher et al, 2015	Phase II, multi-institutional	66, Resectable	56 Gy with Gemcitabine/Cisplatin	Gemcitabine	57.6	69.7	52.6	47.8	68.4	43.5	17.4	14.4	0.99 [.59, 1.65]
Casadei et al, 2015	Phase II, single institution	38, Resectable	54 Gy with Gemcitabine	Gemcitabine	61.1	75.0	63.6	33.3	45.5	13.3	22.4	19.5	1.0 [0.1, 9.82]
Jang et al, 2018	Phase II/III, multi-institution	50, Borderline Resectable	54 Gy with Gemcitabine	CRT, Gemcitabine	63.0	78.3	82.4	33.3	70.6	16.6	21	12	0.51 [0.28, 0.93]
Verstejine et al, 2020	Phase III, multi-institutional	246, Resectable and Borderline	36 Gy with Gemcitabine	Gemcitabine	60.5	72.4	70.8	40.2	66.7	21.7	16	14.3	0.78 [0.58–1.05]

Abbreviations: HR, hazard ratio; N0, node negative; NT, neoadjuvant therapy; R0, negative margins; UFS, up-front surgery.

resections, the ESPAC 1 study called into question the benefits of chemoradiation as adjuvant chemoradiation was associated with a worsened overall survival. Although this trial has been heavily critiqued because of inconsistent dosing and delivery techniques of radiation and use of split course radiation, which is considered an outdated technique, the trial results tempered enthusiasm for radiation therapy.[53] In the neoadjuvant setting, multiple studies have demonstrated improved local control, and improved overall survival associated with pathologic complete response after chemoradiation.[26,54,55]

In the last 6 years, several randomized phase II/III studies have compared neoadjuvant chemoradiation to up-front surgery with adjuvant chemotherapy (**Table 4**). These trials have further demonstrated the neoadjuvant chemoradiation has improved R0 rates and nodal negative disease rates. The most recent and largest of the studies, PREOPANC, observed on subset analysis that the patients with borderline resectable disease treated with neoadjuvant chemoradiation had a significantly improved overall survival compared with up-front surgery (17.6 months vs 13.2 months, HR 0.67 [0.45-0.99] while the patients with resectable disease did not (14.6 months vs 15.6 months, HR: 0.79 [0.54-1.16].[30]

Neoadjuvant chemoradiation improves R0 resections and nodal disease burden in resectable and borderline PDAC, although the survival benefit on is less clear for patients with resectable disease, and may only become evident with longer follow-up.[43] Additional modern, well-controlled randomized trials are needed to determine the efficacy of different fractionation approaches (intensity-modulated radiation therapy vs stereotactic body radiation therapy), and define which patients will most benefit from neoadjuvant chemoradiation.

SUMMARY

The last few decades have revolutionized our understanding and treatment of PDAC. Neoadjuvant therapy has become the preferred treatment approach for patients with operable PDAC however it is still in its nacency and much remains to be understood about the delivery, assessment, and optimization of this treatment approach. Additional studies are needed to evaluate the value of molecular profiling in PDAC, understand the value of adaptive modification of neoadjuvant therapy in response to dynamic changes in biomarker (CA19-9) response, and further define the benefit of radiation therapy. Although PDAC remains a challenging disease to treat, with continued scientific innovation and translational clinical trials, great improvement in outcomes is possible.

DISCLOSURE

The authors have nothing to disclose.

REFERENCES

1. Evans DB, Rich TA, Byrd DR, et al. Connelly JH, Levin B, et al. Preoperative chemoradiation and pancreaticoduodenectomy for adenocarcinoma of the pancreas. Arch Surg 1992;127(11):1335–9.
2. Makary MA, Winter JM, Cameron JL, et al. Pancreaticoduodenectomy in the very elderly. J Gastrointest Surg 2006;10(3):347–56.
3. Winter JM, Brennan MF, Tang LH, et al. Survival after resection of pancreatic adenocarcinoma: results from a single institution over three decades. Ann Surg Oncol 2012;19(1):169–75.

4. Ghaneh P, Kleeff J, Halloran CM, et al. The Impact of Positive Resection Margins on Survival and Recurrence Following Resection and Adjuvant Chemotherapy for Pancreatic Ductal Adenocarcinoma. Ann Surg 2017;269(3):520–9.

5. Grutzmann R, McFaul C, Bartsch DK, et al. No evidence for germline mutations of the LKB1/STK11 gene in familial pancreatic carcinoma. Cancer Lett 2004; 214(1):63–8.

6. Oettle H, Neuhaus P, Hochhaus A, et al. Adjuvant chemotherapy with gemcitabine and long-term outcomes among patients with resected pancreatic cancer: the CONKO-001 randomized trial. J Am Med Assoc 2013;310(14):1473–81.

7. Bilimoria KY, Bentrem DJ, Ko CY, et al. National failure to operate on early stage pancreatic cancer. Ann Surg 2007;246(2):173–80.

8. Fergus J, Nelson DW, Sung M, et al. Pancreatectomy in Stage I pancreas cancer: national underutilization of surgery persists. HPB (Oxford) 2020;22(12):1703–10.

9. Sohal DP, Walsh RM, Ramanathan RK, et al. Pancreatic adenocarcinoma: treating a systemic disease with systemic therapy. J Natl Cancer Inst 2014;106(3):dju011.

10. Rhim AD, Mirek ET, Aiello NM, et al. EMT and dissemination precede pancreatic tumor formation. Cell 2012;148(1–2):349–61.

11. Cunningham D, Allum WH, Stenning SP, et al. Perioperative chemotherapy versus surgery alone for resectable gastroesophageal cancer. N Engl J Med 2006; 355(1):11–20.

12. Primrose JN, Fox RP, Palmer DH, et al. Capecitabine compared with observation in resected biliary tract cancer (BILCAP): a randomised, controlled, multicentre, phase 3 study. Lancet Oncol 2019;20(5):663–73.

13. Conroy T, Hammal P, Hebbar M, et al. Unicancer GI PRODIGE 24/CCTG PA.6 trial: A multicenter international randomized phase III trial of adjuvant mFOLFIRIONX versus gemcitabine in patients wtih resected pancreatic ductal adenocarcinomas. J Clin Oncol 2018;36(Suppl; abstr LABA4001).

14. Wu W, He J, Cameron JL, et al. The impact of postoperative complications on the administration of adjuvant therapy following pancreaticoduodenectomy for adenocarcinoma. Ann Surg Oncol 2014;21(9):2873–81.

15. Merkow RP, Bilimoria KY, Tomlinson JS, et al. Postoperative complications reduce adjuvant chemotherapy use in resectable pancreatic cancer. Ann Surg 2014; 260(2):372–7.

16. Mayo SC, Gilson MM, Herman JM, et al. Management of patients with pancreatic adenocarcinoma: national trends in patient selection, operative management, and use of adjuvant therapy. J Am Coll Surg 2012;214(1):33–45.

17. Conroy T, Desseigne F, Ychou M, et al. FOLFIRINOX versus gemcitabine for metastatic pancreatic cancer. N Engl J Med 2011;364(19):1817–25.

18. Ghaneh P, Palmer DH, Cicconi S, et al. ESPAC-5F: Four-arm, prospective, multicenter, international randomized phase II trial of immediate surgery compared with neoadjuvant gemcitabine plus capecitabine (GEMCAP) or FOLFIRINOX or chemoradiotherapy (CRT) in patients with borderline resectable pancreatic cancer. J Clin Oncol 2020;38(15_suppl):4505.

19. Groot VP, Rezaee N, Wu W, et al. Patterns, Timing, and Predictors of Recurrence Following Pancreatectomy for Pancreatic Ductal Adenocarcinoma. Ann Surg 2017;267(5):936–45.

20. Evans DB, Varadhachary GR, Crane CH, et al. Preoperative gemcitabine-based chemoradiation for patients with resectable adenocarcinoma of the pancreatic head. J Clin Oncol 2008;26(21):3496–502.

21. Sohal D, Duong MT, Ahmad SA, et al. SWOG S1505: Results of perioperative chemotherapy (peri-op CTx) with mfolfirinox versus gemcitabine/nab-paclitaxel

(Gem/nabP) for resectable pancreatic ductal adenocarcinoma (PDA). J Clin Oncol 2020;38(15_suppl):4504.

22. Varadhachary GR, Wolff RA, Crane CH, et al. Preoperative gemcitabine and cisplatin followed by gemcitabine-based chemoradiation for resectable adenocarcinoma of the pancreatic head. J Clin Oncol 2008;26(21):3487–95.

23. Neoptolemos JP, Palmer DH, Ghaneh P, et al. Comparison of adjuvant gemcitabine and capecitabine with gemcitabine monotherapy in patients with resected pancreatic cancer (ESPAC-4): a multicentre, open-label, randomised, phase 3 trial. Lancet 2017;389(10073):1011–24.

24. Versteijne E, Suker M, Groothuis K, et al. Preoperative Chemoradiotherapy Versus Immediate Surgery for Resectable and Borderline Resectable Pancreatic Cancer: Results of the Dutch Randomized Phase III PREOPANC Trial. J Clin Oncol 2020;38(16):1763–73.

25. Tsai S, Christians KK, George B, et al. A Phase II Clinical Trial of Molecular Profiled Neoadjuvant Therapy for Localized Pancreatic Ductal Adenocarcinoma. Ann Surg 2018;268(4):610–9.

26. Wittmann D, Hall WA, Christians KK, et al. Impact of Neoadjuvant Chemoradiation on Pathologic Response in Patients With Localized Pancreatic Cancer. Front Oncol 2020;10:460.

27. Cooper AB, Parmar AD, Riall TS, et al. Does the use of neoadjuvant therapy for pancreatic adenocarcinoma increase postoperative morbidity and mortality rates? J Gastrointest Surg 2015;19(1):80–6, discussion 6-7.

28. Dhir M, Malhotra GK, Sohal DPS, et al. Neoadjuvant treatment of pancreatic adenocarcinoma: a systematic review and meta-analysis of 5520 patients. World J Surg Oncol 2017;15(1):183.

29. Versteijne E, Vogel JA, Besselink MG, et al. Meta-analysis comparing upfront surgery with neoadjuvant treatment in patients with resectable or borderline resectable pancreatic cancer. Br J Surg 2018;105(8):946–58.

30. Eijck CHJV, Versteijne E, Suker M, et al. Preoperative chemoradiotherapy to improve overall survival in pancreatic cancer: Long-term results of the multicenter randomized phase III PREOPANC trial. J Clin Oncol 2021;39(15_suppl):4016.

31. Pancreatic Adenocarcinoma 2021. 2021. Available at: http://www.nccn.org/professionals/physician_gls/pdf/pancreatic.pdf. Accessed February 25, 2021.

32. Iglesias Garcia J, Dominguez-Munoz JE. [Endoscopic ultrasound-guided biopsy for the evaluation of pancreatic tumors]. Gastroenterol Hepatol 2007;30(10):597–601.

33. Eloubeidi MA, Chen VK, Eltoum IA, et al. Endoscopic ultrasound-guided fine needle aspiration biopsy of patients with suspected pancreatic cancer: diagnostic accuracy and acute and 30-day complications. Am J Gastroenterol 2003;98(12):2663–8.

34. Decker C, Christein JD, Phadnis MA, et al. Biliary metal stents are superior to plastic stents for preoperative biliary decompression in pancreatic cancer. Surg Endosc 2011;25(7):2364–7.

35. Aadam AA, Evans DB, Khan A, et al. Efficacy and safety of self-expandable metal stents for biliary decompression in patients receiving neoadjuvant therapy for pancreatic cancer: a prospective study. Gastrointest Endosc 2012;76(1):67–75.

36. Mullen JT, Lee JH, Gomez HF, et al. Pancreaticoduodenectomy after placement of endobiliary metal stents. J Gastrointest Surg 2005;9(8):1094–104, discussion 104-5.

37. Seo DW, Sherman S, Dua KS, et al. Covered and uncovered biliary metal stents provide similar relief of biliary obstruction during neoadjuvant therapy in pancreatic cancer: a randomized trial. Gastrointest Endosc 2019;90(4):602–612 e4.
38. Suk KT, Kim HS, Kim JW, et al. Risk factors for cholecystitis after metal stent placement in malignant biliary obstruction. Gastrointest Endosc 2006;64(4): 522–9.
39. Shimizu S, Naitoh I, Nakazawa T, et al. Predictive factors for pancreatitis and cholecystitis in endoscopic covered metal stenting for distal malignant biliary obstruction. J Gastroenterol Hepatol 2013;28(1):68–72.
40. Nakai Y, Isayama H, Kawakubo K, et al. Metallic stent with high axial force as a risk factor for cholecystitis in distal malignant biliary obstruction. J Gastroenterol Hepatol 2014;29(7):1557–62.
41. Jariwalla NR, Khan AH, Dua K, et al. Management of Acute Cholecystitis during Neoadjuvant Therapy in Patients with Pancreatic Adenocarcinoma. Ann Surg Oncol 2019;26(13):4515–21.
42. Sohal DPS, Duong M, Ahmad SA, et al. Efficacy of Perioperative Chemotherapy for Resectable Pancreatic Adenocarcinoma: A Phase 2 Randomized Clinical Trial. J Am Med Assoc Oncol 2021;7(3):421–7.
43. Cloyd JM, Williams TM. Neoadjuvant Therapy Versus Immediate Surgery for Resectable Pancreas Cancer: Still Open for Debate. Am J Clin Oncol 2020; 43(10):752–4.
44. Rashid NU, Peng XL, Jin C, et al. Purity Independent Subtyping of Tumors (PurIST), A Clinically Robust, Single-sample Classifier for Tumor Subtyping in Pancreatic Cancer. Clin Cancer Res 2020;26:82–92.
45. Aung KL, Fischer SE, Denroche RE, et al. Genomics-Driven Precision Medicine for Advanced Pancreatic Cancer: Early Results from the COMPASS Trial. Clin Cancer Res 2018;24(6):1344–54.
46. Golan T, Hammel P, Reni M, et al. Maintenance Olaparib for Germline BRCA-Mutated Metastatic Pancreatic Cancer. N Engl J Med 2019;381(4):317–27.
47. Wattenberg MM, Asch D, Yu S, et al. Platinum response characteristics of patients with pancreatic ductal adenocarcinoma and a germline BRCA1, BRCA2 or PALB2 mutation. Br J Cancer 2020;122(3):333–9.
48. Murphy JE, Wo JY, Ryan DP, et al. Total Neoadjuvant Therapy With FOLFIRINOX in Combination With Losartan Followed by Chemoradiotherapy for Locally Advanced Pancreatic Cancer: A Phase 2 Clinical Trial. JAMA Oncol 2019;5(7): 1020–7.
49. Kim RY, Christians KK, Aldakkak M, et al. Total Neoadjuvant Therapy for Operable Pancreatic Cancer. Ann Surg Oncol 2021;28(4):2246–56.
50. Boone BA, Steve J, Zenati MS, et al. Serum CA 19-9 response to neoadjuvant therapy is associated with outcome in pancreatic adenocarcinoma. Ann Surg Oncol 2014;21(13):4351–8.
51. Katz MH, Varadhachary GR, Fleming JB, et al. Serum CA 19-9 as a marker of resectability and survival in patients with potentially resectable pancreatic cancer treated with neoadjuvant chemoradiation. Ann Surg Oncol 2010;17(7):1794–801.
52. Tsai S, George B, Wittmann D, et al. Importance of Normalization of CA19-9 Levels Following Neoadjuvant Therapy in Patients With Localized Pancreatic Cancer. Ann Surg 2020;271(4):740–7.
53. Neoptolemos JP, Stocken DD, Friess H, et al. A randomized trial of chemoradiotherapy and chemotherapy after resection of pancreatic cancer. N Engl J Med 2004;350(12):1200–10.

54. He J, Blair AB, Groot VP, et al. Is a Pathological Complete Response Following Neoadjuvant Chemoradiation Associated With Prolonged Survival in Patients With Pancreatic Cancer? Ann Surg 2018;268(1):1–8.
55. Katz MH, Fleming JB, Bhosale P, et al. Response of borderline resectable pancreatic cancer to neoadjuvant therapy is not reflected by radiographic indicators. Cancer 2012;118(23):5749–56.
56. Talamonti MS, Small WJr, Mulcahy MF, et al. A multi-institutional phase II trial of preoperative full-dose gemcitabine and concurrent radiation for patients with potentially resectable pancreatic carcinoma. Ann Surg Oncol 2006;13(2):150–8.
57. Heinrich S, Pestalozzi BC, Schäfer M, et al. Prospective phase II trial of neoadjuvant chemotherapy with gemcitabine and cisplatin for resectable adenocarcinoma of the pancreatic head. J Clin Oncol 2008;26(15):2526–31.
58. Kim EJ, Ben-Josef E, Herman JM, et al. A multi-institutional phase 2 study of neoadjuvant gemcitabine and oxaliplatin with radiation therapy in patients with pancreatic cancer. Cancer 2013;119(15):2692–700.
59. Katz MH, Shi Q, Ahmad SA, et al. Preoperative Modified FOLFIRINOX Treatment Followed by Capecitabine-Based Chemoradiation for Borderline Resectable Pancreatic Cancer: Alliance for Clinical Trials in Oncology Trial A021101. JAMA 2016;151(8):e161137.
60. Murphy JE, Wo JY, Ryan DP, et al. Total Neoadjuvant Therapy With FOLFIRINOX Followed by Individualized Chemoradiotherapy for Borderline Resectable Pancreatic Adenocarcinoma: A Phase 2 Clinical Trial. JAMA Oncol 2018;4(7):963–9.
61. Wei AC, Ou FS, Shi Q, et al. Perioperative Gemcitabine + Erlotinib Plus Pancreaticoduodenectomy for Resectable Pancreatic Adenocarcinoma: ACOSOG Z5041 (Alliance) Phase II Trial. Ann Surg Oncol 2019;26(13):4489–97.
62. Unno M, Motoi F, Matsuyama Y, et al. Randomized phase II/III trial of neoadjuvant chemotherapy with gemcitabine and S-1 versus upfront surgery for resectable pancreatic cancer (Prep-02/JSAP-05). Journal of Clinical Oncology 37(4):189-189. DOI: 10.1200/JCO.2019.37.4_suppl.189.

Evolution of Systemic Therapy in Metastatic Pancreatic Ductal Adenocarcinoma

Mandana Kamgar, MD, MPH*, Sakti Chakrabarti, MD,
Aditya Shreenivas, MD, MS, Ben George, MD

KEYWORDS

- Pancreatic cancer • Adenocarcinoma of the pancreas • Systemic treatment
- Chemotherapy • Evolution

KEY POINTS

- The development of more effective combination chemotherapy has been the main achievement in pancreatic ductal adenocarcinoma within the past decades.
- Despite aggressive multiagent chemotherapy, pancreatic ductal adenocarcinoma outcomes remain poor.
- Targeting tumor metabolism, autophagy, stroma, and cancer cachexia is currently of great interest.
- New approaches to inhibit Kirsten rat sarcoma viral oncogene homologue and its downstream are being explored.

BACKGROUND

Pancreatic ductal adenocarcinoma (PDAC) is a highly aggressive malignancy with the worst prognosis among all gastrointestinal cancers by stage.[1] Several factors contribute to the poor prognosis of PDAC. The presenting symptoms of this cancer are nonspecific, the location is such that cancer cannot be easily detected by physical examination, and there exists no effective screening for this cancer. PDAC, therefore, in the majority of cases (>50%) is diagnosed at an advanced metastatic stage.[2] Even in the early localized stage, and despite aggressive treatment, including multiagent chemotherapy and surgery, 60% or more of the patients experience disease

Division of Hematology and Oncology, Department of Medicine, LaBahn Pancreatic Cancer Program, Medical College of Wisconsin, 9200 West Wisconsin Avenue, Milwaukee, WI 53226, USA
* Corresponding author.
E-mail address: mkamgar@mcw.edu

Surg Oncol Clin N Am 30 (2021) 673–691
https://doi.org/10.1016/j.soc.2021.06.004
1055-3207/21/© 2021 Elsevier Inc. All rights reserved.
surgonc.theclinics.com

recurrence in 3 years or less, with the majority of the recurrences being distant.[3] This signifies that PDAC is a systemic disease with a high tendency for early spread and development of micrometastasis.

The systemic nature of PDAC underscores the importance of systemic therapy in determining the prognosis. However, a vast majority of patients with PDAC exhibit primary resistance or rapidly develop resistance to anticancer drugs, resulting in rapid disease progression despite systemic therapy.[4] The pathobiological underpinnings of PDAC explain the therapeutic refractoriness. Genomic studies of PDAC revealed numerous alterations upregulating various oncogenic pathways in the same tumor that make targeting the cancer-promoting pathways difficult. Integrated profiling of 150 PDAC specimens revealed recurrent somatic mutations in KRAS, TP53, CDKN2A, SMAD4, RNF43, ARID1A, TGFbR2, GNAS, RREB1, and PBRM1.[5] Most of these mutations are not yet targetable. The refractoriness to systemic therapies in PDAC may also be partly attributed to the complex tumor microenvironment that is dominated by dense stroma and immunosuppressive cells,[6,7] which hinders the delivery of drugs to the cancer cells and limits the role of immunotherapy in PDAC.

With limited success with targeted therapy and immunotherapy, cytotoxic chemotherapy remains the mainstream of treatment in metastatic PDAC (mPDAC), the evolution of which will be reviewed in this article. It is notable that, although multiagent chemotherapy improved outcomes in PDAC, many patients might not be able to benefit from such aggressive treatment. PDAC is mostly a disease of the elderly, with a median age at diagnosis of 70 years. Furthermore, the wasting syndrome of cachexia that often accompanies patients with advanced PDAC leads to a rapid deterioration of the performance status, resulting in poor tolerance to aggressive treatment.[8] Therefore, apart from focusing on measures to increase longevity in PDAC, the continuous evaluation of goals of treatment and aggressive supportive care are integral to optimal patient care.

STANDARD SYSTEMIC CHEMOTHERAPY IN METASTATIC PANCREATIC DUCTAL ADENOCARCINOMA
First-Line Chemotherapy

Table 1 summarizes some of the most prominent first-line clinical trials in mPDAC. Single-agent gemcitabine remained the standard first-line treatment of mPDAC for more than a decade, based on a randomized trial reporting a slightly superior median overall survival (mOS) (5.6 months vs 4.4 months) with gemcitabine versus 5-fluorouracil (5-FU) in treatment-naive patients.[9] After years of negative gemcitabine/plus studies,[10] gemcitabine/erlotinib led to improved mOS versus gemcitabine/placebo, although the magnitude of added benefit was small (6.2 months vs 5.9 months).[11] Gemcitabine/erlotinib is therefore not universally adopted, and single-agent gemcitabine remains the most widely used option in patients with PDAC who otherwise do not qualify for more aggressive multiagent chemotherapy.

Currently, folinic acid/5-FU/irinotecan/oxaliplatin (FFX) (FOLFIRINOX) and gemcitabine/nab-paclitaxel (GnP) are the preferred first-line chemotherapy regimens in patients with mPDAC with good performance status (Eastern Cooperative Oncology Group [ECOG] status of 0–1 for FFX and ECOG status of 0–2 for GnP) and without availability of clinical trials. PRODIGE 4 was the phase III trial that showed superior survival with FFX versus gemcitabine (mOS of 11.1 months vs 6.8 months). The MPACT phase III trial showed superiority of GnP over gemcitabine (mOS of 8.5 months vs 6.7 months)[4,12] (see **Table 1**). There is no head-to-head prospective trial comparing

Table 1
Studies evaluating efficacy and safety of first-line chemotherapy in mPDAC

Study (Year)	Trial Phase	Treatment	No.	Median OS (mo)	ORR	Toxicity	Comments
Leading to US Food and Drug Administration approval							
Burris et al,[9] 1997	3	Gemcitabine vs 5-FU	126	5.6 vs 4.4 (P = .002)	5.4% vs 0%	Neutropenia ≥ grade 3: 25.9% vs 4.9% (P < .001)	Survival >12 mo: 18% vs 2%. Clinical benefit response: 23.8% vs 4.8%; (P = .002).
Moore et al,[11] 2007	3	Gemcitabine/erlotinib vs gemcitabine/placebo	569	6.2 vs 5.9 (P = .038)	8.6% vs 8.0%	Higher frequencies of rash, diarrhea, infection, and stomatitis with gemcitabine/erlotinib	One-year survival 23% vs 17%; (P = .023)
Conroy et al,[4] 2011	3	FFX vs gemcitabine	342	11.1 vs 6.8 (P < .001)	31.6% vs 9.4%	Febrile neutropenia 5.4% with FFX	PFS: 6.4 vs 3.3 mo (P < .001)
Von Hoff et al,[12] 2013	3	GnP vs gemcitabine	861	8.5 vs 6.7 (P < .001)	23% vs 7%	Grade ≥ 3 toxicities: neutropenia 38% vs 27%. neuropathy 17% vs 1%.	PFS: 5.5 vs 3.7 mo (P < .001)
Other studies							
Berlin et al,[85] 2002	3	Gemcitabine/bolus 5-FU vs Gemcitabine	322	6.7 vs 5.4 (P = .09).	6.9% vs 5.6%	comparable	PFS 3.4 vs 2.2 mo; (P = .02)
Heinemann et al,[86] 2006	3	Gemcitabine/cisplatin vs gemcitabine	195	7.5 vs 6.0 (P = .15)	10.2% vs 8.2%	Nausea and vomiting 22.2% vs 5.9%; P < .001	PFS 5.3 vs 3.1 mo (P = .053) SD 60.2% vs 40.2%; P < .001
Cunningham et al,[87] 2009	3	Gemcitabine/capecitabine vs gemcitabine	533	7.1 vs 6.2 (P = .08)	19.1% vs 12.4%	Grade ≥ 3 neutropenia 35% vs 22%	PFS: 5.3 vs 3.8 mo (P = .004)
Tempero et al,[88] 2003	2	Gemcitabine 30-min infusion vs FDR	92	5 vs 8 (P = .013)	9% vs 6%	Increased hematologic toxicity with FDR	
Jameson et al,[41] 2019	1b/2	GnPC	25	16.4	71%	Grade ≥3 toxicities: thrombocytopenia (68%), anemia (32%), and neutropenia (24%).	PFS 10.1 mo

Abbreviations: FDR, fixed dose rate; FFX, FOLRIFINOX; GnP, gemcitabine/nab-paclitaxel; GnPC, gemcitabine/nab-paclitaxel, cisplatin; n, number of patients; ORR, objective response rate; SD, stable disease.

FFX with GnP. A meta-analysis of 16 retrospective studies found no difference in OS (hazard ratio, 0.99; 95% confidence interval, 0.84–1.16; $P = .9$) or progression-free survival (PFS) (hazard ratio, 0.88; 95% confidence interval, 0.71–1.1; $P = .26$) between FFX and GnP, although the weighted mOS slightly favored FFX (mean difference, 1.15; 95% confidence interval, 0.08–2.22; $P = .03$).[13]

Until predictive biomarkers of differential response to these regimens are found, the choice of first-line therapy between FFX and GnP largely relies on the physician and/or patient preference and toxicity profiles. Although nausea, vomiting, diarrhea, fatigue, neuropathy, and myelosuppression are more common with FFX, alopecia, skin rash, and fluid overload are more common with GnP.[4,12] Currently, mutations in DNA damage repair genes, such as BRCA1/2 and PALB2, are among the biomarkers predicting potentially improved outcomes with platinum-based therapy (such as FFX or gemcitabine/cisplatin) versus GnP.[14,15] Although not directly comparing FFX with GnP, the phase III NAPOLI-3 trial comparing GnP with NALIRIFOX (liposomal irinotecan [Nal-IRI]/5-FU/LV/oxaliplatin) might set the standard for first-line treatment in patients otherwise qualifying for both regimens (see **Table 3**).

Second-Line Chemotherapy

The survival of patients who receive second-line chemotherapy for mPDAC varies widely. The decision to pursue second-line chemotherapy is influenced by a variety of factors, including the regimen used in the first-line therapy, performance status, comorbidities, and patient preference. Several regimens have shown activity in the gemcitabine-refractory or fluoropyrimidine (FP)-refractory patients, and examples are outlined in **Table 2**.

Treatment after Folinic Acid/5-Fluorauracil/Irinotecan/Oxaliplatin

If FFX was used in the first-line setting and the patient has acceptable performance status without any prohibitive comorbidity, GnP is a reasonable option. The efficacy of GnP in FFX-refractory patients has been evaluated in 2 studies[16,17] (see **Table 2**). In the AGEO prospective cohort study, the overall response rate was 18% and mOS 8.8 months.[17] The other phase II study reported an overall response rate of 13% and mOS 7.6 months.[16] In patients with poor performance status, single-agent gemcitabine or best supportive care are acceptable options.

Treatment after a Gemcitabine-Based Regimen

In patients with PDAC who progressed on first-line gemcitabine-based chemotherapy, the randomized phase III NAPOLI-1 trial demonstrated the superiority of 5-FU/LV/Nal-IRI over 5-FU/LV (mOS of 6.1 months vs 4.2 months)[18] (see **Table 2**). Based on the results of this trial, 5-FU/LV/Nal-IRI received approval from the US Food and Drug Administration as a second-line chemotherapy in the gemcitabine-refractory setting in PDAC with an ECOG status of 0 to 2. Whether 5-FU/LV/Nal-IRI outperforms FOLFIRI (5-FU/LV/irinotecan) has not been evaluated in a randomized study. In a phase II study, the use of FOLFIRI showed comparable efficacy[19] (see **Table 2**). Single-agent FP therapy or supportive care are acceptable options for those with an ECOG status of 2 or greater.

Several oxaliplatin-based regimens have been evaluated in the gemcitabine-refractory setting, including oxaliplatin in combination with a FP,[20–25] gemcitabine,[26] irinotecan,[27] and docetaxel.[28] In the randomized phase III CONKO-003 trial, the OFF regimen (oxaliplatin plus short-term infusional-5-FU/LV) improved survival compared with the best supportive care (mOS of 5.9 months vs 3.3 months).[29] However, a subsequent phase III trial (PANCREOX) with modified-FOLFOX6 versus

Table 2
Key studies evaluating efficacy of second-line chemotherapy in mPDAC

Study (Year)	Design/phase	Treatment	No.	Median OS (mo)	Median PFS (mo)	Comments
Progression after gemcitabine-based regimens						
Wang-Gillam et al,[18] 2016[a]	3	5-FU/LV/Nal-IRI vs 5-FU/LV	417	6.1 vs 4.2 (P = .012)	3.1 vs 1.5 (P < .001).	Nal-IRI alone arm was also tested and was found inferior
Oettle et al,[29] 2014	3	OFF vs 5-FU/LV	160	5.9 vs 3.3 (P = .01)	2.9 vs 2 (HR = 0.68; P = .019)	Grade 1/2 neurotoxicity (38.2% vs 7.1%)
Gill et al,[21] 2016	3	mFOLFOX6 vs 5-FU/LV	108	6.1 vs 9.9 (P = .02)	3.1 vs 2.9 (P = .99)	Withdrawal from study due to adverse events (20% vs 2%) Percentage who received subsequent lines of therapy (7% vs 25%)
Kim et al,[35] 2018	2	mFFX	39	8.5	3.8	ORR 10.3% Grade 3–4 neutropenia in 40%
Xiong et al,[25] 2008	2	XELOX	41	6	2.5	6-mo and 1-y survival rates were 44% and 21%
Katopodis et al,[32] 2011	2	Docetaxel/ capecitabine	31	6.3	2.4	ORR 10%
Zaniboni et al,[19] 2012	2	FOLFIRI	50	5	3.2	ORR 8% 6-mo survival rate was 32%.
Sawada et al,[89] 2020	Retrospective	mFFX	104	7	3.9	ORR 10.6%
Progression after FP-based regimens						
Mita et al,[16] 2019	2	GnP	30	7.6	3.8	ORR 13.3%
Demols et al,[26] 2006	2	GEMOX	31	6	Not reported	Partial response in 22.6%

(continued on next page)

Table 2
(continued)

Study (Year)	Design/phase	Treatment	No.	Median OS (mo)	Median PFS (mo)	Comments
Hosein et al,[34] 2013	2	Nab-paclitaxel	19	7.3	1.7	
Ettrich et al,[28] 2016	2	Docetaxel/oxaliplatin	44	10.1	1.8	ORR 15.9%
Portal et al,[17] 2015	Multicenter cohort	GnP	57	8.8	5.1	ORR 17.5%. Grade 3–4 toxicities in 40% (neutropenia 12.5% and neurotoxicity 12.5%)

Abbreviations: FFX, FOLFIRINOX (5-FU/leucovorin/oxaliplatin/irinotecan); FOLFIRI, 5-FU/leucovorin/irinotecan; FOLFOX, 5-FU/leucovorin/oxaliplatin; GEMOX, gemcitabine/oxaliplatin; GnP, gemcitabine/nab-paclitaxel; HR, hazard ratio; LV, leucovorin; mFFX, modified-FOLFIRINOX; mFOLFOX6, modified-FOLFOX6; Nal-IRI, liposomal irinotecan; OFF, oxaliplatin/5-FU/leucovorin; ORR, overall response rate; XELOX, capecitabine/oxaliplatin.
[a] Led to approval by the US Food and Drug Administration.

infusional-5-FU/LV showed inferior mOS with modified-FOLFOX6 (mOS of 9.9 months vs 6.1 months; P = .02). Although a clear explanation of this discrepant result is lacking, possible explanations are: increased proportion of patients receiving treatment after progression in the 5-FU/LV arm compared with the modified-FOLFOX-6 arm (25% vs 7%), and higher proportion of grade 3/4 adverse events with modified-FOLFOX-6 (63% vs 11%), resulting in a 10-fold higher withdrawal rate (20% vs 2%). Furthermore, the mOS in the 5-FU/LV arm was better in the PANCREOX trial than in the corresponding arms of CONKO-003 and NAPOLI-1 trials.

A phase III study is not available to compare the efficacy of FOLFOX versus FOLFIRI in patients with gemcitabine-refractory disease. A randomized phase II study comparing FOLFOX versus FOLFIRI in the second-line setting reported a similar 6-month OS rate—27% with FOLFIRI and 30% with FOLFOX.[30] A meta-analysis of second-line trials concluded that the combination of FP plus irinotecan significantly improved both PFS and OS, whereas oxaliplatin-based combinations modestly improved PFS but not OS.[31] Other agents with activity in the patient population with gemcitabine-refractory disease are docetaxel plus oxaliplatin,[28] docetaxel plus capecitabine,[32] gemcitabine and oxaliplatin,[26] single-agent FP (eg, S1),[33] and nab-paclitaxel,[34] as outlined in **Table 2**.

Multiple retrospective studies have explored the role of FFX or one of its modified versions in the gemcitabine-refractory setting (see **Table 2**). A phase II study evaluated the role of modified-FFX (with omission of 5-FU bolus and 25% dose reductions of infusional-5-FU, irinotecan, and oxaliplatin) in patients with gemcitabine-refractory disease with an ECOG status of 0 to 1 and without prohibitive symptoms and reported a mOS of 8.5 months[35] (see **Table 2**). The study did not use prophylactic growth factor support and encountered frequent grade 3 to 4 neutropenia (40%). Use of modified-FFX is, therefore, a potential option in this setting, although prophylactic growth factor support, close follow-up, and further modifications of the regimen based on tolerance would be warranted.

Fig. 1 depicts the algorithm of management of mPDAC at the authors' institution.

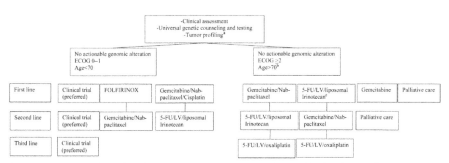

Fig. 1. Treatment algorithm for PDAC management at the Medical College of Wisconsin.[a] If actionable alterations found, treatment is adjusted accordingly: BRCA1/2 or PALB2 or other homologous recombinant deficient tumors: FOLFIRINOX or gemcitabine cisplatin followed by maintenance PARP inhibitor; mismatch repair deficient, or high tumor mutational burden: immunotherapy (pembrolizumab vs nivolumab/ipilumumab); KRAS wild type: targeted therapy based on detected mutations (such as BRAF V600E or EGFR) or fusions (such as NTRK, ALK, reactive oxygen species-1, RET, or NRG-1). [b]Regimens might need to be started at a lower dose with increase based on tolerance. [c]Used for those otherwise able to tolerate doublet regimen, but with baseline peripheral neuropathy.

EMERGING CONCEPTS IN CHEMOTHERAPY
Maintenance Therapy

Chemotherapy

The role of maintenance therapy is increasingly being explored in the management of mPDAC. The phase II PANOPTIMOX trial evaluated the efficacy and safety of 6 months of FFX (arm A), 4 months of FFX, followed by maintenance 5-FU/LV (arm B), and alternating regimen of FOLFIRI.3 and gemcitabine every 2 months until progression (arm C). The PFS rate at 6 months (the primary end point for this study) in arms A, B, and C was 47%, 44%, and 34%, respectively, showing the effectiveness of arms A and B, but not C. The median PFS and OS in arms A and B, respectively, were 6.3 and 5.7 months and 10.1 and 11.2 months.[36]

Similarly, the efficacy and safety of gemcitabine maintenance after GnP have been studied in a prospective observational study in older adults (>70 years) with locally advanced or mPDAC.[37] After the maximum 3 months of GnP, 31 patients were treated with gemcitabine. The disease control rate at 6 months was 61%, the median PFS 6.4 months, and the mOS was 13.1 months. None of the patients experienced grade 3 neuropathy.

Poly ADP ribose polymerase inhibition

In the subgroups of patients with germline BRCA1/2 mutation, olaparib, a poly ADP ribose polymerase inhibition (PARP) inhibitor, is now an established maintenance option. In the phase III POLO trial, PDAC patients with germline BRCA mutation treated with 16 or more weeks of platinum without progression were randomized to olaparib or placebo. Maintenance olaparib was associated with improved median PFS (7.4 vs 3.8 months; hazard ratio, 0.53; $P = .004$), but not mOS,[38] without health-related quality of life deterioration.[39] Backed by preclinical data,[40] 2 trials are testing the value of the addition of immune checkpoint inhibitors to maintenance PARP-inhibitor (**Table 3**). Other ongoing trials in the maintenance setting, are evaluating the role of other PARP inhibitors or testing the value of other biomarkers for PARP sensitivity (see **Table 3**). Whether maintenance treatment can be expanded beyond chemotherapy and PARP inhibition is also tested (see **Table 3**).

New Combinations of Old Drugs

Other than GnP and FFX combinations, the chemotherapy drug components of these regimens have been tested as part of multiple other combination regimens.

A phase Ib/II study evaluated the safety and response rate of gemcitabine/nab-paclitaxel/cisplatin (GnPC) as first-line chemotherapy in 25 mPDAC patients. Although this study did not meet its primary end point ($\geq$25% complete response) and was associated with 2 treatment-associated deaths, it showed a high response rate of 71% with a disease control rate of 88% and mOS of 16.4 months.[41] GnPC is currently being further evaluated in mPDAC (see **Table 3**).

The safety and tolerability of a liposomal irinotecan (Nal-IRI)/5-FU/LV/oxaliplatin (NALIRIFOX regimen) was tested in a phase I/II study. The results of this study showed acceptable tolerability, with an overall response rate of 34.4%, a median PFS of 9.2 months, and an mOS of 12.6 months.[42] NALIRIFOX is currently being compared with GnP in the phase III NAOPOLI-3 study (see **Table 3**).

A single-center, single-arm phase II study showed acceptable safety of FOLFOX-A (FOLFOX plus nab-paclitaxel) as first-line chemotherapy in mPDAC (NCT02080221). A phase II study is comparing this regimen with GnP (see **Table 3**).

Table 3
Selected clinical trials in advanced PDAC

Approach/Target	Population	Drug	Additional Treatment	Treatment Setting	Study Phase	Study Identifier
Maintenance						
PARP	BRCA1/2 or PALB2 Mutated (germline or somatic)[a]	Rucaparib		Maintenance	2	NCT03140670
PARP + PD-1	BRCA1/2 mutated (germline)[a]	Olaparib	+ Pembrolizumab	Maintenance	2	NCT04548752
PARP + (PD-1 or CTLA-4)	Platinum sensitive[a]	Niraparib	+ (Nivolumab or ipilimumab)	Maintenance	1/2	NCT03404960
PARP	BRCAness + or KRAS-mutated[a]	Olaparib	Or selumetinib/durvalumab or FOLFIRI[b]	Maintenance	2	NCT04348045
PD-1 + vitamin D pathway	After best possible response[c]	Pembrolizumab	+ (Paricalcitol or placebo)	Maintenance	2	NCT03331562
New combinations of old drugs	A-PDAC	NALIRIFOX[d]	Or GnP	First line	3	NCT04083235
	A-PDAC	GnPC		First line	2	NCT03915444
	A-PDAC	FOLFOX-A[e]	Or GnP	First line	2	NCT04151277
KRAS[f]						
RNA interference	LA-PDAC	siG12D-LODER/GnP	Or GnP	First line	2	NCT01676259
SOS-1	Advanced solid tumor	BI 1701963	+/− trametinib	Late line	1	NCT04111458
Autophagy inhibition/downstream of KRAS						
ERK + autophagy		LY3214996	+/− Hydroxychloroquine	Second or third line	2	NCT04386057
Autophagy + MEK + PD-L1	KRAS-mutated, including PDAC cohort	Hydroxychloroquine	+ Cobimetinib + atezolizumab	Late line	1/2	NCT04214418
Autophagy + MEK		Hydroxychloroquine	+ Trametinib	Beyond first line	1	NCT03825289
Autophagy + MEK	KRAS-mutated	Hydroxychloroquine	+ Binimetinib	Beyond first line	1	NCT04132505

(continued on next page)

Table 3
(continued)

Approach/Target	Population	Drug	Additional Treatment	Treatment Setting	Study Phase	Study Identifier
Stromal reprogramming						
Connective tissue growth factor	LA-PDAC	+/– Pamrevlumab	GnP		3	NCT03941093
VDR		Paricalcitol	+ GnP	First line	1/2	NCT03520790
VDR		Paricalcitol	+ GnPC	First line	2	NCT03415854
VDR		Paricalcitol[g]	+ (GnP or GnPC)		2	NCT04054362
VDR + PD-1		Paricalcitol	+ (GnPC) + Nivolumab	First line	2	NCT02754726
VDR + autophagy		Paricalcitol	+ GnP + hydroxychloroquine	First line	2	NCT04524702
Vitamin A derivative		+/-ATRA	GnP	First line	2	NCT04241276
Metabolism						
KGDH/PDH		+/– CPI-613	FFX	First line	3	NCT03504423
GAPDH	FFX-refractory	GP-2250	+ gemcitabine	Second line	1/2	NCT03854110
Asparagine		Eryaspase	+ (GnP or FOLFIRI or 5-FU/LV/Nal-IRI)	Second line	3	NCT03665441
Asparagine		Eryaspase	+ mFFX	First line	1	NCT04292743
Tyrosine		SM-88	Or (gemcitabine or FP)	Late line	2/3	NCT03512756
Tyrosine		SM-88	FFX or GnP	First line	3	NCT04229004

Abbreviations: A-PDAC, Advanced-PDAC; ATRA, All-trans retinoic acid; BRCA, breast cancer gene; CTLA-4, cytotoxic T-lymphocyte-associated protein 4; EGFR, epidermal growth factor receptor; ERK, extracellular signal-regulated kinase; FFX, FOLFIRINOX; GAPDH, glyceraldehyde-3-phosphate dehydrogenase; GnP, gemcitabine/nab-paclitaxel; GnPC, gemcitabine/nab-paclitaxel/cisplatin; KGDH, ketoglutarate dehydrogenase; LA-PDAC, locally advanced PDAC; MEK, Mitogen/Extracellular signal-regulated Kinase; PALB2, Partner and Localizer of BRCA2; PARP, Poly ADP ribose polymerase; PD-1, Programmed cell death protein 1; PDAC, pancreatic ductal adenocarcinoma; PDH, pyruvate dehydrogenase; PD-L1, Programmed death-ligand 1; SOS-1, Son of sevenless homolog-1; VDR, vitamin D receptor.

a After stable-disease ≥4 mo on platinum-based therapy.

b BRCAness receives olaparib, KRAS-mutated is randomized to FOLFIRI or selumetinib/durvalumab.

c Best possible response: initial stable disease or partial response ≥2 mo with no more shrinkage of ≥30% on scan.

d 5-FU/LV/Nal-IRI/oxaliplatin.

e 5-FU/LV/oxaliplatin/nab-paclitaxel.

f Excluding KRAS(G12 C) studies.

g Paricalcitol added to GnP or GnPC after stable disease or progression on these regimens.

SYSTEMIC THERAPY BEYOND CHEMOTHERAPY

Currently, there are multiple agents in different stages of development in the management of mPDAC. Some of the most promising examples are summarized in **Table 3** and further discussed in this section.

Kirsten Rat Sarcoma Viral Oncogene Homologue

Kirsten rat sarcoma viral oncogene homologue (KRAS) mutations are known to be the most important driver mutations in PDAC. Unfortunately, KRAS inhibition has remained an elusive target in this disease space. In PDAC, KRAS most frequently mutates at codon 12 (98%).[43] The success of the KRAS(G12C) inhibitor, AMG 510, in heavily pretreated lung cancers harboring KRAS(G12C) mutations,[44] a rare mutation in PDAC (<2%), has brought back enthusiasm to the field of KRAS-based systemic therapy in PDAC.

Targeting Kirsten rat sarcoma viral oncogene homologue

siG12D-LODER is a degradable miniature implant with the ability to be inserted endoscopically in the tumor, releasing small interfering RNA targeting KRAS(G12). A phase I/IIa study using siG12D-LODER plus chemotherapy in the first-line setting in patients with locally advanced PDAC showed acceptable toxicity and efficacy of this combination. The mOS with the combination was 15.1 months with a disease control rate of 83% (10/12). A phase II study is further evaluating the efficacy of this combination (see **Table 3**).

BI 1701963 is a small molecule with the ability to inhibit KRAS activation, and with enhanced tumor efficacy when combined with agents targeting downstream of KRAS.[45] A phase I study is evaluating the maximum tolerated dosage of BI 1701963, alone or in combination with trametinib (see **Table 3**).

Targeting autophagy and downstream of Kirsten rat sarcoma viral oncogene homologue

Autophagy is a process that allows cellular waste recovery and increases the ability of a tumor to sustain metabolic needs in difficult tumor conditions.[46] KRAS-mutated cells are increasingly dependent on autophagy.[47] Hydroxychloroquine, an indirect autophagy inhibitor, alone or in combination with chemotherapy, did not show promising antitumor activity in PDAC.[48,49] MEK or ERK inhibition is shown to increase the dependency of PDAC on autophagy.[50,51] Furthermore, both MEK and autophagy inhibition are connected with proimmunogenic effect, with the ability to enhance the efficacy of checkpoint inhibitors in cancer.[52,53] Currently, multiple studies are evaluating the role of hydroxychloroquine in combination with different MEK or ERK inhibitors ± checkpoint inhibitors (see **Table 3**).

Stroma

Up to 90% of the tumor volume in PDAC may consist of dense desmoplastic stroma[54] that interferes with the drug delivery to the cancer.[55] Depleting this physical barrier, therefore, seems an obvious opportunity to improve chemotherapy efficacy in PDAC. Meddling with the stroma is challenging, however, because it seems to have both tumor-promoting and tumor-retaining functions.[56]

Stromal depletion

Hyaluronic acid (HA) is a glycosaminoglycan rich in the tumor stroma, and its abundance is associated with decreased delivery of the drugs to the tumor.[57] Depletion of HA by pegylated human hyaluronidase (PEGPH20) in HA-rich tumors in the preclinical setting showed improved chemotherapy delivery.[57] Results of a phase I/II study in an HA-rich unselected population showed PEGPH20/FFX to be inferior to FFX.[58] Also, in a phase III trial in HA-high selected patients, PEGPH20/GnP did not improve OS or PFS compared with GnP.[59]

The overexpression of sonic hedgehog (shh) in PDAC is associated with increased stromal desmoplasia.[60] A phase I/II study of vismodegib (a shh inhibitor)/gemcitabine versus gemcitabine showed no clinical benefit to the combination.[61] Saridegib, another shh inhibitor plus gemcitabine, was found to be inferior to gemcitabine (NCT01130142).

Stromal normalization

Vitamin D receptor is abundantly expressed in the PDAC stroma. Calcipotriol, a vitamin D receptor ligand, can result in stromal remodeling, decreased fibrosis and inflammation, and improved chemotherapeutic response.[62] Paricalcitol, a synthetic vitamin D receptor ligand, is currently being tested in multiple studies in first-line mPDAC (see **Table 3**). Preliminary results of the paricalcitol/GnPC/nivolumab phase II study among the first 10 evaluated patients showed an encouraging response rate of 80%,[63] and further enrollment in this study is ongoing. A small phase I study is evaluating the safety and efficacy of paricalcitol/5-FU/LV/Nal-IRI in the second-line setting in advanced PDAC (NCT03883919).

All-trans retinoic acid, a vitamin A derivative with an established role in the treatment of promyelocytic leukemia, has been repurposed recently as an agent with the potential for stromal reprogramming.[64] A phase Ib study established safety of the All-trans retinoic acid/GnP combination.[64] A phase IIb study is further exploring the efficacy of All-trans retinoic acid/GnP (see **Table 3**).

Connective tissue growth factor is linked to increased stromal fibrosis and tumor aggressiveness.[65] FG-3019 (pamrevlumab), a monoclonal antibody against connective tissue growth factor, is associated with decreased fibrosis, tumor growth, and metastasis.[66] A phase I/II study evaluated the safety and efficacy of pamrevlumab/GnP in patients with locally advanced PDAC (NCT02210559). Compared with GnP alone, pamrevlumab/GnP was associated with higher rates of surgical resection (33% vs 8%) without additional serious adverse events.[66] A phase III study is further exploring the value of this combination (see **Table 3**).

Tumor Metabolism

Mitochondrial metabolism

Altered mitochondrial metabolism is a well-known characteristic of cancer cells.[67] CPI-613 (devimistat) is a lipoate analogue that by inactivating 2 of the crucial enzymes in the Krebs cycle acts as a tumor-specific antimitochondrial metabolism agent.[68,69] In a phase I study, a combination of CPI-613 with modified FFX (mFFX) was well-tolerated with a 61% objective response rate.[70] The efficacy of CPI-613/mFFX versus FFX in first-line mPDAC is being tested in a phase III study (NCT03504423). Although accrual of the intended 500 patients to this study has completed, final results are pending. CPI-613/GnP was also found to be safe, with an objective response rate of 50% in a phase I study.[71]

BMP31510 is a ubidecarenone (oxidized coenzyme Q10) using a nanodispersion mechanism to preferentially deliver the drug to the cancer cells. BMP31510 can shift the tumor metabolism away from lactate dependency, resulting in reactive oxygen species formation and apoptosis.[72] The safety of BMP31510 in advanced solid tumors, alone or in combination with different chemotherapy agents, was shown in a phase I study (NCT01957735). A phase II study showed the safety of BMP31510/gemcitabine in patients with advanced PDAC.[73]

GP-2250 is an oxathiazine derivative with the ability to inhibit GAPDH (glyceraldehyde-3-phosphate dehydrogenase), a rate-limiting enzyme in aerobic glycolysis.[74] It causes the production of reactive oxygen species and induces apoptosis preferentially in the cancer cells. The safety of GP-2250/gemcitabine combination is being studied (see **Table 3**).

Amino acid metabolism
Tumor cells (vs normal human cells) preferentially depend on external supply of nonessential amino acids, such as asparagine and tyrosine, for their survival.[75]

L-Asparaginase can deplete the plasma asparagine and lead to cancer cell death.[76] Two ongoing studies are evaluating the safety and efficacy of different combinations of eryaspase, L-asparaginase encapsulated in red blood cells, in PDAC (see **Table 3**). ADI-PEG 20 is a pegylated form of arginine deaminase (another arginine depleting enzyme). A phase I/Ib study showed safety of ADI-PEG 20/GnP combination with a response rate of 45.5% in the 5 patients treated in the first-line setting.[77]

SM-88 (racemetyrosine) is a dysfunctional tyrosine designed to interfere with the tyrosine metabolism in cancer cells. When combined with physiologic, but subtherapeutic, doses of methoxalen, phenytoin, and sirolimus, the uptake of SM-88 by cells can be enhanced and the defense of tumor cells against oxidative stress and host immunity can be exploited.[78] A phase I study in advanced solid tumors established the safety of this combination.[78] Its role in PDAC is being tested in later phase studies (see **Table 3**).

Cachexia and Sarcopenia

Cachexia and sarcopenia are common findings among patients with PDAC and are associated with a worse prognosis, as well as worse treatment tolerance.[79]

Anamorelin, a ghrelin receptor agonist, is an agent with the ability to improve cancer-related cachexia through multiple mechanisms, including stimulation of growth hormone secretion.[80] Anamorelin is approved in Japan for treating cancer cachexia.[81] Approval for advanced gastrointestinal cancers was based on a multicenter, single-arm study in Japan, which showed improvement of anorexia, and gain of lean body mass and weight with daily anamorelin.[82] Anamorelin/chemotherapy in PDAC is planned to be tested in a phase II clinical trial.

IL-1α, a proinflammatory cytokine, is associated with cachexia and muscle atrophy.[83] The safety of bermikimab (IL-1α antagonist)/5-FU/LV/Nal-IRI was established in a phase I trial.[84] Although bermikimab did not lead to weight or lean body mass gain, it was associated with a decrease in the C-reactive protein level and improvement of quality of life and physical, emotional, and functional well-being. Among the 18 evaluable patients, 22% had partial response and 72% had stable disease.[84] This combination is further planned to be studied as part of a phase I/II trial.

SUMMARY

With the improvement of care of patients with PDAC, including the availability of more effective multiagent chemotherapies, the 5-year survival for PDAC increased slightly from 3% to 4% in 1975% to 1989% to 10% in 2010 to 2016.[1] While exploring new combinations of currently existing chemotherapeutic agents could lead to more flexibility in choosing treatments based on the comorbidities of patients, this approach would be incomplete unless coupled with the use of predictive biomarkers to personalize treatment options. Emerging nonchemotherapeutic approaches, such as targeting KRAS and its downstream, evaluating tumor metabolism, stromal reprogramming, and autophagy are all promising avenues being actively explored in the management of advanced PDAC.

CLINICS CARE POINTS

- All patients with PDAC should be encouraged to participate in clinical trials when feasible.
- Systemic chemotherapy should be administered with close monitoring and dose modifications personalized to patient genotype and phenotype.
- Aggressive supportive care along with multi-agent chemotherapy is integral to optimizing clinical outcome in patients with PDAC.

DISCLOSURE

M. Kamgar, A. Shreenivas, S. Chakrabarti: none to disclose. B. George: Consultation for Celgene, Ipsen, Foundation Medicine, Bristol-Myer Squibb, Exelixis, Taiho Oncology, and Roche/Genentech; Research funding from Roche/Genentech, Boehringer Ingelheim, Tolero, Toray, NGM Biopharmaceuticals, Helix BioPharma, Hutchison Medipharma.

REFERENCES

1. American Cancer Society. Cancer facts & figures 2021. Atlanta: American Cancer Society; 2021.
2. Siegel RL, Miller KD, Fuchs HE, et al. Cancer statistics, 2021. CA Cancer J Clin 2021;71(1):7–33.
3. Barnes CA, Aldakkak M, Christians KK, et al. Radiographic patterns of first disease recurrence after neoadjuvant therapy and surgery for patients with resectable and borderline resectable pancreatic cancer. Surgery 2020;168(3):440–7.
4. Conroy T, Desseigne F, Ychou M, et al. FOLFIRINOX versus gemcitabine for metastatic pancreatic cancer. N Engl J Med 2011;364(19):1817–25.
5. Raphael BJ, Hruban RH, Aguirre AJ, et al. Integrated genomic characterization of pancreatic ductal adenocarcinoma. Cancer Cell 2017;32(2):185–203.e113.
6. Huber M, Brehm CU, Gress TM, et al. The immune microenvironment in pancreatic cancer. Int J Mol Sci 2020;21(19).
7. Thomas D, Radhakrishnan P. Tumor-stromal crosstalk in pancreatic cancer and tissue fibrosis. Mol Cancer 2019;18(1):14.
8. Biswas AK, Acharyya S. Understanding cachexia in the context of metastatic progression. Nat Rev Cancer 2020;20(5):274–84.
9. Burris HA 3rd, Moore MJ, Andersen J, et al. Improvements in survival and clinical benefit with gemcitabine as first-line therapy for patients with advanced pancreas cancer: a randomized trial. J Clin Oncol 1997;15(6):2403–13.
10. Rahib L, Fleshman JM, Matrisian LM, et al. Evaluation of pancreatic cancer clinical trials and benchmarks for clinically meaningful future trials: a systematic review. JAMA Oncol 2016;2(9):1209–16.
11. Moore MJ, Goldstein D, Hamm J, et al. Erlotinib plus gemcitabine compared with gemcitabine alone in patients with advanced pancreatic cancer: a phase III trial of the National Cancer Institute of Canada Clinical Trials Group. J Clin Oncol 2007;25(15):1960–6.

12. Von Hoff DD, Ervin T, Arena FP, et al. Increased survival in pancreatic cancer with nab-paclitaxel plus gemcitabine. N Engl J Med 2013;369(18):1691–703.

13. Pusceddu S, Ghidini M, Torchio M, et al. Comparative effectiveness of gemcitabine plus Nab-Paclitaxel and FOLFIRINOX in the first-line setting of metastatic pancreatic cancer: a systematic review and meta-analysis. Cancers (Basel) 2019;11(4).

14. O'Reilly EM, Lee JW, Zalupski M, et al. Randomized, multicenter, phase II trial of gemcitabine and cisplatin with or without veliparib in patients with pancreas adenocarcinoma and a germline BRCA/PALB2 mutation. J Clin Oncol 2020; 38(13):1378–88.

15. Park W, Chen J, Chou JF, et al. Genomic methods identify homologous recombination deficiency in pancreas adenocarcinoma and optimize treatment selection. Clin Cancer Res 2020;26(13):3239–47.

16. Mita N, Iwashita T, Uemura S, et al. Second-line gemcitabine plus nab-paclitaxel for patients with unresectable advanced pancreatic cancer after first-line FOLFIRINOX failure. J Clin Med 2019;8(6).

17. Portal A, Pernot S, Tougeron D, et al. Nab-paclitaxel plus gemcitabine for metastatic pancreatic adenocarcinoma after Folfirinox failure: an AGEO prospective multicentre cohort. Br J Cancer 2015;113(7):989–95.

18. Wang-Gillam A, Li CP, Bodoky G, et al. Nanoliposomal irinotecan with fluorouracil and folinic acid in metastatic pancreatic cancer after previous gemcitabine-based therapy (NAPOLI-1): a global, randomised, open-label, phase 3 trial. Lancet 2016;387(10018):545–57.

19. Zaniboni A, Aitini E, Barni S, et al. FOLFIRI as second-line chemotherapy for advanced pancreatic cancer: a GISCAD multicenter phase II study. Cancer Chemother Pharmacol 2012;69(6):1641–5.

20. Berk V, Ozdemir N, Ozkan M, et al. XELOX vs. FOLFOX4 as second line chemotherapy in advanced pancreatic cancer. Hepatogastroenterology 2012;59(120): 2635–9.

21. Gill S, Ko YJ, Cripps C, et al. PANCREOX: a randomized phase III study of fluorouracil/leucovorin with or without oxaliplatin for second-line advanced pancreatic cancer in patients who have received gemcitabine-based chemotherapy. J Clin Oncol 2016;34(32):3914–20.

22. Lee K, Bang K, Yoo C, et al. Clinical outcomes of second-line chemotherapy after progression on nab-paclitaxel plus gemcitabine in patients with metastatic pancreatic adenocarcinoma. Cancer Res Treat 2020;52(1):254–62.

23. Pelzer U, Schwaner I, Stieler J, et al. Best supportive care (BSC) versus oxaliplatin, folinic acid and 5-fluorouracil (OFF) plus BSC in patients for second-line advanced pancreatic cancer: a phase III-study from the German CONKO-study group. Eur J Cancer 2011;47(11):1676–81.

24. Pointet AL, Tougeron D, Pernot S, et al. Three fluoropyrimidine-based regimens in routine clinical practice after nab-paclitaxel plus gemcitabine for metastatic pancreatic cancer: An AGEO multicenter study. Clin Res Hepatol Gastroenterol 2020;44(3):295–301.

25. Xiong HQ, Varadhachary GR, Blais JC, et al. Phase 2 trial of oxaliplatin plus capecitabine (XELOX) as second-line therapy for patients with advanced pancreatic cancer. Cancer 2008;113(8):2046–52.

26. Demols A, Peeters M, Polus M, et al. Gemcitabine and oxaliplatin (GEMOX) in gemcitabine refractory advanced pancreatic adenocarcinoma: a phase II study. Br J Cancer 2006;94(4):481–5.

27. Cantore M, Rabbi C, Fiorentini G, et al. Combined irinotecan and oxaliplatin in patients with advanced pre-treated pancreatic cancer. Oncology 2004;67(2):93–7.

28. Ettrich TJ, Perkhofer L, von Wichert G, et al. DocOx (AIO-PK0106): a phase II trial of docetaxel and oxaliplatin as a second line systemic therapy in patients with advanced pancreatic ductal adenocarcinoma. BMC Cancer 2016;16:21.

29. Oettle H, Riess H, Stieler JM, et al. Second-line oxaliplatin, folinic acid, and fluorouracil versus folinic acid and fluorouracil alone for gemcitabine-refractory pancreatic cancer: outcomes from the CONKO-003 trial. J Clin Oncol 2014; 32(23):2423–9.

30. Yoo C, Hwang JY, Kim JE, et al. A randomised phase II study of modified FOLFIRI.3 vs modified FOLFOX as second-line therapy in patients with gemcitabine-refractory advanced pancreatic cancer. Br J Cancer 2009; 101(10):1658–63.

31. Sonbol MB, Firwana B, Wang Z, et al. Second-line treatment in patients with pancreatic ductal adenocarcinoma: a meta-analysis. Cancer 2017;123(23): 4680–6.

32. Katopodis O, Polyzos A, Kentepozidis N, et al. Second-line chemotherapy with capecitabine (Xeloda) and docetaxel (Taxotere) in previously treated, unresectable adenocarcinoma of pancreas: the final results of a phase II trial. Cancer Chemother Pharmacol 2011;67(2):361–8.

33. Sudo K, Yamaguchi T, Nakamura K, et al. Phase II study of S-1 in patients with gemcitabine-resistant advanced pancreatic cancer. Cancer Chemother Pharmacol 2011;67(2):249–54.

34. Hosein PJ, de Lima Lopes G Jr, Pastorini VH, et al. A phase II trial of nab-paclitaxel as second-line therapy in patients with advanced pancreatic cancer. Am J Clin Oncol 2013;36(2):151–6.

35. Kim JH, Lee SC, Oh SY, et al. Attenuated FOLFIRINOX in the salvage treatment of gemcitabine-refractory advanced pancreatic cancer: a phase II study. Cancer Commun (Lond) 2018;38(1):32.

36. Dahan L, Phelip JM, Malicot KL, et al. FOLFIRINOX until progression, FOLFIRINOX with maintenance treatment, or sequential treatment with gemcitabine and FOLFIRI.3 for first-line treatment of metastatic pancreatic cancer: a randomized phase II trial (PRODIGE 35-PANOPTIMOX). J Clin Oncol 2018;36(15_suppl): 4000.

37. Petrioli R, Torre P, Pesola G, et al. Gemcitabine plus nab-paclitaxel followed by maintenance treatment with gemcitabine alone as first-line treatment for older adults with locally advanced or metastatic pancreatic cancer. J Geriatr Oncol 2020;11(4):647–51.

38. Golan T, Hammel P, Reni M, et al. Maintenance olaparib for germline BRCA-mutated metastatic pancreatic cancer. N Engl J Med 2019;381(4):317–27.

39. Hammel P, Kindler HL, Reni M, et al. Health-related quality of life in patients with a germline BRCA mutation and metastatic pancreatic cancer receiving maintenance olaparib. Ann Oncol 2019;30(12):1959–68.

40. Stewart RA, Pilie PG, Yap TA. Development of PARP and immune-checkpoint inhibitor combinations. Cancer Res 2018;78(24):6717–25.

41. Jameson GS, Borazanci E, Babiker HM, et al. Response rate following albumin-bound paclitaxel plus gemcitabine plus cisplatin treatment among patients with advanced pancreatic cancer: a phase 1b/2 pilot clinical trial. JAMA Oncol 2020;6(1):125–32.

42. Wainberg Z, Bekaii-Saab T, Boland P, et al. LBA-1 first-line liposomal irinotecan + 5 fluorouracil/leucovorin + oxaliplatin in patients with pancreatic ductal

adenocarcinoma: long-term follow-up results from a phase 1/2 study. Ann Oncol 2020;31:S241.

43. Bryant KL, Mancias JD, Kimmelman AC, et al. KRAS: feeding pancreatic cancer proliferation. Trends Biochem Sci 2014;39(2):91–100.

44. Hong DS, Fakih MG, Strickler JH, et al. KRAS(G12C) inhibition with sotorasib in advanced solid tumors. N Engl J Med 2020;383(13):1207–17.

45. Gerlach D, Gmachl M, Ramharter J, et al. Abstract 1091: BI-3406 and BI 1701963: potent and selective SOS1::KRAS inhibitors induce regressions in combination with MEK inhibitors or irinotecan. Cancer Res 2020;80(16 Supplement): 1091.

46. Guo JY, White E. Autophagy, metabolism, and cancer. Cold Spring Harb Symp Quant Biol 2016;81:73–8.

47. Yang S, Wang X, Contino G, et al. Pancreatic cancers require autophagy for tumor growth. Genes Dev 2011;25(7):717–29.

48. Wolpin BM, Rubinson DA, Wang X, et al. Phase II and pharmacodynamic study of autophagy inhibition using hydroxychloroquine in patients with metastatic pancreatic adenocarcinoma. Oncologist 2014;19(6):637–8.

49. Karasic TB, O'Hara MH, Loaiza-Bonilla A, et al. Effect of gemcitabine and nab-paclitaxel with or without hydroxychloroquine on patients with advanced pancreatic cancer: a phase 2 randomized clinical trial. JAMA Oncol 2019;5(7):993–8.

50. Bryant KL, Stalnecker CA, Zeitouni D, et al. Combination of ERK and autophagy inhibition as a treatment approach for pancreatic cancer. Nat Med 2019;25(4): 628–40.

51. Kinsey CG, Camolotto SA, Boespflug AM, et al. Protective autophagy elicited by RAF–>MEK–>ERK inhibition suggests a treatment strategy for RAS-driven cancers. Nat Med 2019;25(4):620–7.

52. Baumann D, Hagele T, Mochayedi J, et al. Proimmunogenic impact of MEK inhibition synergizes with agonist anti-CD40 immunostimulatory antibodies in tumor therapy. Nat Commun 2020;11(1):2176.

53. Autophagy inhibition synergizes with immunotherapy in pancreatic cancer. Cancer Discov 2020;10(6):760.

54. Neesse A, Algul H, Tuveson DA, et al. Stromal biology and therapy in pancreatic cancer: a changing paradigm. Gut 2015;64(9):1476–84.

55. Netti PA, Berk DA, Swartz MA, et al. Role of extracellular matrix assembly in interstitial transport in solid tumors. Cancer Res 2000;60(9):2497–503.

56. Hosein AN, Brekken RA, Maitra A. Pancreatic cancer stroma: an update on therapeutic targeting strategies. Nat Rev Gastroenterol Hepatol 2020;17(8):487–505.

57. Thompson CB, Shepard HM, O'Connor PM, et al. Enzymatic depletion of tumor hyaluronan induces antitumor responses in preclinical animal models. Mol Cancer Ther 2010;9(11):3052–64.

58. Ramanathan RK, McDonough SL, Philip PA, et al. Phase IB/II randomized study of FOLFIRINOX plus pegylated recombinant human hyaluronidase versus FOLFIRINOX alone in patients with metastatic pancreatic adenocarcinoma: SWOG S1313. J Clin Oncol 2019;37(13):1062–9.

59. Van Cutsem E, Tempero MA, Sigal D, et al. Randomized phase III trial of pegvorhyaluronidase alfa with Nab-paclitaxel plus gemcitabine for patients with hyaluronan-high metastatic pancreatic adenocarcinoma. J Clin Oncol 2020; 38(27):3185–94.

60. Bailey JM, Swanson BJ, Hamada T, et al. Sonic hedgehog promotes desmoplasia in pancreatic cancer. Clin Cancer Res 2008;14(19):5995–6004.

61. Catenacci DV, Junttila MR, Karrison T, et al. Randomized phase Ib/II study of gemcitabine plus placebo or vismodegib, a hedgehog pathway inhibitor, in patients with metastatic pancreatic cancer. J Clin Oncol 2015;33(36):4284–92.

62. Sherman MH, Yu RT, Engle DD, et al. Vitamin D receptor-mediated stromal reprogramming suppresses pancreatitis and enhances pancreatic cancer therapy. Cell 2014;159(1):80–93.

63. Borazanci EH, Jameson GS, Borad MJ, et al. A phase II pilot trial of nivolumab (N) + albumin bound paclitaxel (AP) + paricalcitol (P) + cisplatin (C) + gemcitabine (G) (NAPPCG) in patients with previously untreated metastatic pancreatic ductal adenocarcinoma (PDAC). J Clin Oncol 2018;36(4_suppl):358.

64. Kocher HM, Basu B, Froeling FEM, et al. Phase I clinical trial repurposing all-trans retinoic acid as a stromal targeting agent for pancreatic cancer. Nat Commun 2020;11(1):4841.

65. Charrier A, Brigstock DR. Regulation of pancreatic function by connective tissue growth factor (CTGF, CCN2). Cytokine Growth Factor Rev 2013;24(1):59–68.

66. Aikawa T, Gunn J, Spong SM, et al. Connective tissue growth factor-specific antibody attenuates tumor growth, metastasis, and angiogenesis in an orthotopic mouse model of pancreatic cancer. Mol Cancer Ther 2006;5(5):1108–16.

67. Vander Heiden MG, Cantley LC, Thompson CB. Understanding the Warburg effect: the metabolic requirements of cell proliferation. Science 2009;324(5930):1029–33.

68. Zachar Z, Marecek J, Maturo C, et al. Non-redox-active lipoate derivates disrupt cancer cell mitochondrial metabolism and are potent anticancer agents in vivo. J Mol Med (Berl) 2011;89(11):1137–48.

69. Stuart SD, Schauble A, Gupta S, et al. A strategically designed small molecule attacks alpha-ketoglutarate dehydrogenase in tumor cells through a redox process. Cancer Metab 2014;2(1):4.

70. Alistar A, Morris BB, Desnoyer R, et al. Safety and tolerability of the first-in-class agent CPI-613 in combination with modified FOLFIRINOX in patients with metastatic pancreatic cancer: a single-centre, open-label, dose-escalation, phase 1 trial. Lancet Oncol 2017;18(6):770–8.

71. Alistar AT, Morris B, Harrison L, et al. A single-arm, open-label, phase I study of CPI-613 (Devimistat) in combination with gemcitabine and nab-paclitaxel for patients with locally advanced or metastatic pancreatic adenocarcinoma. J Clin Oncol 2020;38(15_suppl):4635.

72. Niewiarowska AA, Lucius DM, Sarangarajan R, et al. A phase 2 clinical investigation of BPM31510-IV (Ubidecarenone) in patients with advanced pancreatic cancer. Ann Oncol 2018;29(suppl_8):viii205–70.

73. Kundranda MN, Propper D, Ritch PS, et al. Phase II trial of BPM31510-IV plus gemcitabine in advanced pancreatic ductal adenocarcinomas (PDAC). J Clin Oncol 2020;38(4_suppl):723.

74. Braumann C, Buchholz M, Stiller BM, et al. Metabolism-based GP-2250 in combination with gemcitabine as a novel approach to pancreatic cancer: a mouse xenograft study. J Clin Oncol 2020;38(15_suppl):e16750.

75. Bachet JB, Gay F, Marechal R, et al. Asparagine synthetase expression and phase I study with L-asparaginase encapsulated in red blood cells in patients with pancreatic adenocarcinoma. Pancreas 2015;44(7):1141–7.

76. Schrek R, Dolowy WC, Ammeraal RN. L-asparaginase: toxicity to normal and leukemic human lymphocytes. Science 1967;155(3760):329–30.

77. Lowery MA, Yu KH, Kelsen DP, et al. A phase 1/1B trial of ADI-PEG 20 plus nab-paclitaxel and gemcitabine in patients with advanced pancreatic adenocarcinoma. Cancer 2017;123(23):4556–65.
78. Stega J, Noel MS, Vandell AG, et al. A first-in-human study of the novel metabolism-based anti-cancer agent SM-88 in subjects with advanced metastatic cancer. Invest New Drugs 2020;38(2):392–401.
79. Susanto B, Hariyanto TI, Kurniawan A. The impact of sarcopenia on chemotherapy toxicity and survival rate among pancreatic cancer patients who underwent chemotherapy: a systematic review and meta-analysis. Ann Oncol 2020; 31(suppl_6):S1287–318.
80. Garcia JM, Polvino WJ. Pharmacodynamic hormonal effects of anamorelin, a novel oral ghrelin mimetic and growth hormone secretagogue in healthy volunteers. Growth Horm IGF Res 2009;19(3):267–73.
81. Wakabayashi H, Arai H, Inui A. The regulatory approval of anamorelin for treatment of cachexia in patients with non-small cell lung cancer, gastric cancer, pancreatic cancer, and colorectal cancer in Japan: facts and numbers. J Cachexia Sarcopenia Muscle 2021;12(1):14–6.
82. Hamauchi S, Furuse J, Takano T, et al. A multicenter, open-label, single-arm study of anamorelin (ONO-7643) in advanced gastrointestinal cancer patients with cancer cachexia. Cancer 2019;125(23):4294–302.
83. Fearon KC, Glass DJ, Guttridge DC. Cancer cachexia: mediators, signaling, and metabolic pathways. Cell Metab 2012;16(2):153–66.
84. Hendifar AE, Kim S, Tighiouart M, et al. A phase I study of nanoliposomal irinotecan and 5-fluorouracil/folinic acid in combination with interleukin-1-alpha antagonist for advanced pancreatic cancer patients with cachexia (OnFX). J Clin Oncol 2020;38(15_suppl):4634.
85. Berlin JD, Catalano P, Thomas JP, Kugler JW, Haller DG, Benson AB. 3rd. Phase III study of gemcitabine in combination with fluorouracil versus gemcitabine alone in patients with advanced pancreatic carcinoma: Eastern Cooperative Oncology Group Trial E2297. J Clin Oncol 2002;20(15):3270–5.
86. Heinemann V, Quietzsch D, Gieseler F, Gonnermann M, Schonekas H, Rost A, et al. Randomized phase III trial of gemcitabine plus cisplatin compared with gemcitabine alone in advanced pancreatic cancer. J Clin Oncol 2006;24(24): 3946–52.
87. Cunningham D, Chau I, Stocken DD, Valle JW, Smith D, Steward W, et al. Phase III randomized comparison of gemcitabine versus gemcitabine plus capecitabine in patients with advanced pancreatic cancer. J Clin Oncol 2009;27(33):5513–8.
88. Tempero M, Plunkett W, Ruiz Van Haperen V, Hainsworth J, Hochster H, Lenzi R, et al. Randomized phase II comparison of dose-intense gemcitabine: thirty-minute infusion and fixed dose rate infusion in patients with pancreatic adenocarcinoma. J Clin Oncol 2003;21(18):3402–8.
89. Sawada M, Kasuga A, Mie T, Furukawa T, Taniguchi T, Fukuda K, et al. Modified FOLFIRINOX as a second-line therapy following gemcitabine plus nab-paclitaxel therapy in metastatic pancreatic cancer. BMC Cancer 2020;20(1):449.

Precision Medicine and Pancreatic Cancer

Ben George, MD

KEYWORDS

- Precision medicine • Pancreatic cancer • Comprehensive genomic profiling

KEY POINTS

- Precision therapeutics in pancreatic cancer is rapidly evolving.
- Germline alterations in DNA damage repair genes currently constitute the most prevalent actionable therapeutic target in pancreas cancer.
- Germline and somatic mismatch repair deficiency status as well as various somatic fusion kinases serve as predictive biomarkers in a small subset of patients with pancreas cancer.
- Harnessing the advances in molecular translation and bioinformatics is pivotal to realizing the promise of precision therapeutics in pancreas cancer.

INTRODUCTION

Pancreatic ductal adenocarcinoma (PDAC) is expected to become the second leading cause of cancer-related mortality in the United States, second only to lung cancer in the next decade.[1] Therapeutic advances over the last decade have translated into a survival benefit that can at best be characterized as modest. The improvement in survival over the years can be attributed to improvements in multimodality oncologic care (surgery, radiotherapy, and systemic chemotherapy), aggressive supportive care, and delivery of therapy to more patients. Furthermore, identification of predictive biomarkers, improved understanding of the tumor microenvironment (TME) as well as the tumor/host immune interactions in PDAC have increased therapeutic opportunities for a subset of patients. Our evolving understanding about the molecular biology of PDAC highlights its complexity, the marked challenges in translating scientific discoveries, and the urgent need to realize the promise of precision therapeutics.

Evolution of PDAC

It has been proposed that PDAC develops in a stepwise fashion, through a sequence of genetic alterations, with a relatively gradual evolutionary trajectory since these alterations are acquired independently.[1–6] However, the identification of clonally expanded precursor lesions that do not belong to the tumor lineage and a clinical phenotype that

Division of Hematology and Oncology, Medical College of Wisconsin, 9200 W. Wisconsin Avenue, Milwaukee, WI 53226, USA
E-mail address: bgeorge@mcw.edu
Twitter: @bengeorge1974 (B.G.)

Surg Oncol Clin N Am 30 (2021) 693–708
https://doi.org/10.1016/j.soc.2021.06.008
1055-3207/21/© 2021 Elsevier Inc. All rights reserved.
surgonc.theclinics.com

demonstrates aggressive metastatic potential argue against that theory.[3,7-10] Notta and colleagues performed an in-depth analysis of over 100 whole genomes from purified primary and metastatic PDACs using novel informatics tools, with a focus on DNA copy number (CN) changes, their associated rearrangements from tumor-enriched genomes, and mutational phenomena linked to rapid tumor progression, to reconcile these disparate theories.[11] They concluded that (i) most mutations accumulate when these tumors are still diploid, suggesting that a prolonged preneoplastic phase (assuming preneoplastic cells are diploid) predates the onset of invasive disease and that CN events are crucial for transformation; (ii) CN changes from chromothripsis appeared to be clonal (suggesting that such events were sustained early in tumorigenesis) and transformative; (iii) some PDACs may not progress through a linear series of PanIN lesions; and (iv) if chromothripsis were indeed the transforming event in some PDACs, a single event could confer a cell with both invasive and metastatic properties, suggesting a short latency period between invasion and metastasis.

Molecular Pathogenesis

A variety of precursor lesions have been described in the pancreas. These include pancreatic intraepithelial neoplasia (PanIN), intraductal papillary mucinous neoplasms (IPMNs), and mucinous cystadenomas (MCNs).[12] PanIN gives rise to conventional ductal adenocarcinomas and they are 13- to 100-fold more common than those arising from an IPMN or MCN.[13] IPMNs are macroscopically visible cystic neoplasms that arise in the mucin-producing main pancreatic duct or one of its branches, whereas MCNs are macroscopically visible cystic neoplasms that do not communicate with the pancreatic duct system.

Many key experimental and epidemiologic observations suggest that PDAC is a genetic disease: (i) several somatic alterations have been recurrently identified in PDAC and many of these have also been identified in precursor lesions[2,4,6]; (ii) PDACs are known to aggregate in some families, and the genetic basis for a subset of these have been well described[14-17]; and (iii) genetically engineered mouse models can recapitulate the full spectrum of pancreatic carcinogenesis and metastasis as seen in humans.[18-20]

Historically, 4 major driver genes have been described in the development and progression of PDAC—1 oncogene (KRAS) and 3 tumor suppressor genes (CDKN2A, TP53, and SMAD4). KRAS is thought to be constitutively activated in 92% to 100% of patients with pancreatic cancer, whereas TP53, SMAD4, and CDKN2A have been reported to be inactivated in 74% to 83%, 31% to 33%, and 35% to 75% of patients, respectively.[21-24] Although these individual genes play a pivotal role in pancreatic carcinogenesis, the recognition that concerted involvement of multiple signaling pathways or cellular processes led to pancreatic carcinogenesis was the basis for early systematic attempts at identifying core pathways and processes involved in PDAC development.[23] Such attempts improved our understanding of PDAC pathogenesis substantially, however, the translated gain in therapeutic improvement was modest at best.

The overall dismal outcome associated with PDACs, the lack of reliable predictive biomarkers to guide therapy, and the significant inter/intratumoral heterogeneity emphasize the need for a unique, "tumor-specific," summative, biologic footprint that offers consistent prognostic and/or predictive information. Major advances in technology and bioinformatics have refined attempts at generating "expression signatures" or "tumor profiles" that reflect tumor-specific genotypic and/or phenotypic information, in a granular fashion. Large-scale attempts have been made to generate genomic, epigenomic, transcriptomic, and proteomic profiles of PDAC, with the goal to identify distinct prognostic and predictive signatures; some of the key attempts have been listed in **Table 1**.

Predictive biomarkers

Various consensus guidelines recommend germline testing for all patients with PDAC and somatic testing for all patients with advanced PDAC. Both germline and somatic genomic profiling will identify a subset of patients with driver genomic alterations with predictive relevance for systemic therapies. The therapeutic relevance of these biomarkers—both germline and somatic is explored in the following:

DNA Damage Repair in PDAC

DNA damage is a common event and several distinct repair mechanisms work to preserve genomic integrity in both normal and malignant cells.[27] DNA double-strand breaks (DSB) bear the greatest risk of provoking genomic instability, and DNA damage

Table 1
Large-scale attempts have been made to generate genomic, epigenomic, transcriptomic, and proteomic profiles of PDAC, with the goal to identify distinct prognostic and predictive signatures

Author, Publication Year	N	Methodology	Discovery
Jones et al,[23] 2008	24	Exome sequencing	Core set of 12 cellular signaling pathways and processes
Collison et al,[25] 2011	2 data sets	Transcriptomic profiling	i. Three subtypes—classical, quasimesenchymal (QM-PDA), and exocrine-like ii. Prognostic value of subtypes
Biankin et al,[22] 2012	99	Whole genome sequencing, CNV analysis	i. 16 significant mutated genes ii. Frequent and diverse somatic aberrations in genes involved in axon guidance (SLIT/ROBO signaling)
Moffitt et al,[26] 2015	206	Transcriptomic profiling	i. Basal and classical tumor subtypes ii. Normal and activated stromal subtypes iii. Prognostic and predictive value of the subtypes
Waddell et al,[24] 2015	100	Whole genome sequencing, CNV analysis	i. Four subtypes—stable, locally rearranged, scattered, and unstable ii. Predictive value of unstable subtype to platinum-based chemotherapy
Bailey et al,[21] 2016	456	Whole genome sequencing, deep exome sequencing, CNV analysis, transcriptomic profiling	i. Four subtypes—squamous, pancreatic progenitor, immunogenic, and aberrantly differentiated endocrine exocrine ii. Identified 32 recurrently mutated genes grouped into 10 pathways

Abbreviations: CNV, copy number variation.

repair (DDR) pathways are pivotal to preserving genomic integrity. Failure of DDR after endogenous and/or exogenous insults can lead to accumulation of genomic defects, structural aberrations, malignant transformation of cells, cancer progression, and resultant synthetic lethality to DNA damaging agents, which can be exploited therapeutically.[27]

DDR gene mutations in PDAC can be germline or somatic. In about 3.9% to 13.5% of patients with apparently sporadic PDAC, DDR gene mutations can be detected in the germline (with negative family history of cancer) because of incomplete penetration.[28–31]

Most of the DDR genes mutated in PDAC are involved in the homologous recombination (HR) pathway. Genetic, epigenetic, or post-translational alterations in these genes lead to a homologous recombination deficient (HRD) phenotype with biological and therapeutic implications in HRD-dependent tumor lineages (breast, prostate, ovarian, and pancreas cancers).[32] DNA damaging cytotoxic therapies (like platinum agents) can crosslink purine bases on the DNA, thereby interrupting DNA transcription, stall replication, cause DSBs, and elicit synthetic lethality in HRD cancer cells.[33]

A recent publication explored the prognostic and predictive relevance of homologous recombination DNA damage response (HR-DDR) gene mutations in 820 PDAC patients enrolled in the Know Your Tumor (KYT) program. Patients were categorized based on clinical stage (resected vs advanced disease), and therapy received (platinum-based therapy vs being platinum naïve). Comprehensive genomic profiling results and longitudinal clinical outcomes were available for all patients.[34] HRD-causing germline or somatic mutations were grouped into 3 categories based on known or suspected platinum responsiveness—(i) BRCA1/2 or PALB2; (ii) ATM/ATR/ATRX; or (iii) BAP1, BARD1, BRIP1, CHEK1/2, RAD50/51/51B, or FANCA/C/D2/E/F/G/L. Patients with advanced HRD PDAC had a worse outcome than patients with HR-proficient (HRP) PDAC if they were not treated with platinum-based chemotherapy, underpinning their negative prognostic impact and platinum susceptibility (median overall survival [mOS]: HRD 0.76 years vs HRP 1.13 years, $P = .1535$). In-line platinum treatment prolonged mOS in the HRD patients (n = 53) compared with the HRP patients (n = 258) (mOS: HRD 2.37 years vs HRP 1.45 years; $P = .000072$; HR, 0.44, 95% CI 0.29–0.66). The mOS positively correlated with an increasing number of HR-related mutations and was independent of the line of treatment. Similarly, several smaller retrospective series have confirmed the platinum sensitivity associated with HRD PDAC as summarized in **Table 2**.

Poly ADP-ribose Polymerase Inhibitors in HRD PDAC

The role poly–ADP-ribose polymerase (PARP)-1 was first characterized in single-stranded break repair through base excision but it is now well-accepted as also participating in DSB repair, stalled replication fork sensing, and in the recruitment of DNA repair proteins at DNA damage sites.[40] As PARP1/2 are pivotal enzymes involved in HR-mediated DSB repair in most cancer cells, targeting these enzymes in HRD tumors exploits the cancer cell vulnerabilities and underpins the principle of synthetic lethality.[40] Several small trials had demonstrated modest activity with single-agent PARP inhibitors in HRD PDAC (summarized in **Table 3**) until the unequivocally positive data from the phase III POLO trial.[41] Patients with centrally confirmed germline BRCA1/BRCA2-mutated advanced PDAC (N = 154) who demonstrated stability or response to frontline platinum-based chemotherapy ($\geq$16 weeks) were randomly assigned to maintenance olaparib or placebo in a 3:2 fashion. The primary endpoint of median PFS was significantly longer with olaparib than placebo (7.4 months vs 3.8 months; HR, 0.53%; 95% [CI], 0.35–0.82; $P = .004$). At the interim analysis, with

Table 2
Several retrospective studies have confirmed the platinum sensitivity associated with HRD PDAC

Author/Publication Year/Ref	N	Mutations	Therapy	mPFS	mOS
Wattenberg et al,[35] 2020	78 HRD -26 HRP - 52	BRCA1, BRCA2, PALB2	Platinum-containing any therapy	HRD + platinum: 10.1 m HRP + platinum: 6.9 m	HRD + platinum: 24.6 m HRP + platinum: 18.8 m
Pishvaian et al,[34] 2019	443 HRD-72 HRP- 371	BRCA1/2, PALB2, ATM, ATR, ATRX, BAP1, BARD1, BRIP1, CHEK1/2, RAD50/51/51B, FANCA/C/D2/E/F/G/L	Platinum containing vs Platinum naive	First-line: HRD + platinum (n = 53): 13.7 m HRP + platinum (n = 268): 8.2 m Second-line: HRD + platinum (n = 28): 8.6 m HRP + platinum (n = 103): 4.1 m	HRD + platinum (n = 53): 2.37 y HRD-platinum (n = 19): 0.76 y HRP + platinum (n = 258): 1.45 y HRP-platinum (n = 113): 1.13 y
Palacio et al,[36] 2019	40	gBRCA2 BRCA2 BRCA1 POLE gRAD51 C gMUTYH	FOLFIRINOX	HRD + platinum- 18.5 m HRP + platinum - 6.9 m	11.5 m
Sehdev et al,[37] 2018	36 HRD-12	BRCA1/2, PALB2, MSH2, FANCF	FOLFIRINOX	NA	HRD: 14 m HRP: 5 m
Kondo et al,[38] 2018	28 HRD-13	BRCA1/2, PALB2, ATM, ATR, CHEK2	Platinum containing therapy	HRD + platinum - 20.8 m HRP + platinum - 1.7 m	NA
Golan et al,[39] 2014	43	BRCA1/2	Platinum containing vs Platinum naive	NA	HRD + platinum (n = 22): 22 m HRD + non-platinum (n = 21): 9 m

Abbreviations: PFS, progression free survival; mPFS, median Progression Free Survival.

Table 3
Several small trials demonstrated modest activity with single-agent PARP inhibitors in HRD PDAC

Author/Publication Year/Reference	Design	N	Mutations	Line of Therapy	Therapy	mPFS	mOS
O'Reilly et al,[42] 2020	Phase II	Total: 50	gBRCA1 gBRCA2 gPALB2	First-line	Cisplatin Gemcitabine ± Veliparib	GCV – 10.1 m GC -9.7 m	GCV – 15.5 GC -16.4
O'Reilly et al,[43] 2018	Phase I	Total: 17 HRD - 9 HRP - 7 Unknown - 1	gBRCA1/2	First-line	Cisplatin Gemcitabine Veliparib		HRD: 23.3 m HRP: 11 m
Shroff et al,[44] 2018	Phase II	19	gBRCA1/2 sBRCA1/2	≥ Second-line	Rucaparib		
Lowery et al,[45] 2018	Phase II	16 HRD -9 HRP-7	gBRCA1/2	≥Second-line	Veliparib	1.7 m	3.1 m
Kaufman et al,[46] 2015	Phase II	23	gBRCA1/2	≥Second-line	Olaparib	9.8 m	

Abbreviations: GC, gemcitabine cisplatin; GCV, gemcitabine cisplatin velipaib.

data maturity of 46%, there was no difference in mOS between the olaparib and pla-cebo groups (mOS, 18.9 months vs 18.1 months; HR, 0.91; 95% CI, 0.56–1.46; $P = .68$). Among patients with measurable disease at baseline, the response rate— assessed by blinded central review—was 23% in the olaparib group and 12% in the placebo group (OR, 2.30; 95% CI, 0.89–6.76). The median duration of response was 24.9 months versus 3.7 months in the olaparib and placebo groups, respectively, with 22.1% of the patients in the olaparib group remaining progression-free at 2 years versus 9.6% of patients in the placebo. Furthermore, the health-related quality of life, based on the European Organization for Research and Treatment of Cancer Quality of Life Questionnaire, was similar between the 2 groups (between-group difference, −2.47 points; 95% CI, −7.27 to 2.33). The incidence of grade 3 or higher adverse events was 40% in the Olaparib group and 23% in the placebo group. Although these data are practice changing, it is important to note that only 7.5% of the 3315 patients screened for entry in the POLO trial had a germline *BRCA* mutation limiting the appli-cability of these data to only to a small proportion of patients with advanced PDAC. Furthermore, presence of a germline BRCA1/2 mutation in PDAC does not automat-ically confer sensitivity to a PARPi. Both somatic genetic alterations as well as epige-netic modifications have been shown to functionally restore HR-DDR and revert the HRD phenotype in ovarian cancer; resistance mechanisms to PARPi need to be further explored in PDAC. The sensitivity of PDACs with somatic BRCA mutations to PARPi also needs further exploration. Available data seem to indicate that in tumor lineages that are BRCA dependent (breast, prostate, ovarian, and pancreas cancers), somatic BRCA mutations may confer sensitivity to PARPi contingent on the overall genomic instability caused by the alteration.[32] In addition, a substantial minority ($\sim$18%) of the potentially eligible patients had disease progression during platinum-based chemotherapy before trial entry highlighting the fact that platinum sensitivity in BRCA1/2-mutated PDAC is not universal. The development of more nuanced, in silico prediction algorithms, make help better patient selection for such biomarker-enriched therapeutic strategies. Finally, the additive value of PARP inhibi-tors in combination with or after a platinum-based regimen is questionable and response predictors in this clinical setting are lacking. PARP inhibitors can increase immune response and induce PD-L1 expression. Nonetheless, whether this estab-lishes a synergistic axis between PARP and immune checkpoint inhibition in HRD PDAC remains unclear.

Microsatellite Instability

The mismatch repair (MMR) system is composed of several genes (MSH2, MSH3, MSH6, PMS1, MLH1, and PMS2) playing a pivotal role in error repair during DNA repli-cation. A defective MMR system leads to random mutations occurring in small repet-itive elements referred to as microsatellite instability (MSI).[47] MSI high (MSI-H) or dMMR is a rare occurrence in PDAC with a frequency of approximately 1% and most of these patients (83%–100%; 5 of 6 and 7 of 7) are found to have Lynch syn-drome.[48,49] Tumors with dMMR have enhanced expression of mutation-associated neoantigens, strong expression of immune checkpoint ligands, and have been shown to benefit from immune checkpoint inhibitors (CPIs) with improved survival.[50] In an analysis of 833 PDAC patients who underwent next-generation sequencing (NGS), 7 were found to have dMMR (0.8%).[48] Among 5 patients who received a PD-1 or PDL-1 inhibitor, 4 had stable disease or durable response. The benefit of single-agent pembrolizumab, a PD-1 inhibitor was further evaluated in a phase 2 trial of dMMR solid tumors—the study included 2 PDAC patients.[50] These results have led to a current recommendation by NCCN to use pembrolizumab as second-line therapy in patients with dMMR or MSI-H PDAC. In addition, in May 2017, immune CPI pembrolizumab was granted tumor site agnostic approval by the US Food and Drug Administration (FDA) for adult and pediatric patients with unresectable or metastatic cancer, which would be identified as dMMR/MSI-H.

Other Predictive Biomarkers

Somatic driver mutations are universal in PDAC and are dominated by KRAS, P53, SMAD4, and CDKN2A. Activating mutations in KRAS are detected in more than 90% of PDAC patients with codon 12 mutations being most frequent.[51] KRAS encodes a small GTPase, which acts as a transducer-effector, cooperating with cell surface receptor tyrosine kinases.[52] Once triggered, it activates different intracellular pathways involved in carcinogenesis, such as proliferation and cell migration, evasion of the immune system, and inhibition of apoptosis. Although many therapeutic efforts have been made to target the function of mutated KRAS oncoprotein, they have been unsuccessful in substantially modifying PDAC prognosis. Although several agents targeting KRAS-downstream pathways (eg, mitogen-activated protein kinase or MEK inhibitors) have been tested alone or in combination with standard cytotoxic therapies and epidermal growth factor receptor (EGFR) inhibitors in advanced PDAC, there are no positive trials.[53] The clinical ineffectiveness of these targeted therapies despite good biologic plausibility can be attributed to the adaptive reactivation of MAPK signaling and multiple pathway redundancies.

A small subgroup of patients with a relatively rare KRAS mutation—KRAS G12C—appear to benefit from a novel inhibitor of KRAS G12C—AMG510. A recently reported phase 1 trial that investigated the role of AMG 510 enrolled 12 patients with PDAC harboring KRAS G12C—one partial response was noted while more than 80% of patients demonstrated stable disease.[54] MRTX849, a potent and specific inhibitor of KRAS G12C, demonstrated robust in vitro activity against KRAS G12C and was used to treat 2 patients with metastatic PDAC whose disease was refractory to multiple lines of therapy.[55] Both patients experienced a partial response after 3 cycles of therapy. This target may have a relatively low clinically impact in Caucasian patients with PDAC because of the rarity of KRAS G12C mutation (1%–2% of patients with PDAC), it will be of tremendous significance in selected patient populations like Japanese where the mutation is seen in about 60% of patients with PDAC.[56]

The minority of PDAC patients with wild-type (WT) KRAS (6%–10%) represent a distinct phenotype, demonstrating an enrichment of therapeutically actionable kinases like Neuregulin 1 (NRG1) rearrangements, NTRK fusion, anaplastic lymphoma kinase (ALK) rearrangements, and ROS.[57,58] Singhi and colleagues analyzed a cohort of 3594 PDACs and reported that kinase fusions were one of the most frequent putative driver alterations in KRAS WT PDACs.[58] They found specific kinase fusions in FGFR2 (12 cases), RAF (7 cases), ALK (5 cases), RET (4 cases), MET (2 cases), NTRK1 (2 cases), ERBB4 (1 case), and FGFR3 (1 case), representing about 7.6% of genetic alterations of all KRAS WT PDAC. In most fusion genes, a serine/threonine kinase or tyrosine kinase catalytic domain was fused to an oligomerization domain, which may represent a mutual mechanism of activation. All these kinase fusions were mutually exclusive, and, like BRAF, they were not present in PDACs with KRAS alterations.

NRG1 rearrangement confers susceptibility to ERBB inhibitors and anti-EGFR antibodies with several patients demonstrating a short-lived partial response to afatinib an EGFR inhibitor.[57,59] In addition, zenocutuzumab (MCLA-128), a bispecific HER-2, −3 antibody is being evaluated in advanced solid tumors with documented *NRG1* gene fusions, including a specific PDAC cohort (NCT02912949).

Neurotrophic tyrosine receptor kinase *(NTRK)* fusion is rare in PDAC—identified in less than 1% of tumors—and results in constitutive activation of *RAS*- and *AKT*-signaling pathways.[60] Partial responses have been reported in response to entrectinib (a potent *TRK* and *ROS1* inhibitor), and larotrectinib, a highly selective *TRK* inhibitor. Next-generation *NTRK* inhibitors are being evaluated in solid tumors with an *NTRK* fusion.[61,62]

ALK gene translocations are a rare event in PDAC. In a comprehensive genomic profiling effort that analyzed over 3500 patients, Singhi and colleagues detected an ALK gene translocation in 5 patients (0.16%).[58] Four of the 5 patients were treated with one or more ALK inhibitors after prior exposure to standard cytotoxic therapy and 3 demonstrated durable stable disease as the best outcome.[58]

BRAF gene mutations are typically mutually exclusive of KRAS mutations representing another genetic alteration in the KRAS WT cohort and account for approximately 3% of somatic mutations in PDAC.[63,64] Of the 18 BRAF-mutant PDAC patients identified in the "KYT" program, 2 were treated with a dabrafenib/trametinib (BRAF/MEK-inhibition) combination and one of the patients (BRAF V600E mutation) had a sustained response to the combination.[65] Another patient with concurrent KRAS G12A and BRAF K601N mutations failed to respond to the treatment. Clinical response as measured by biochemical (CA19-9 decline) and radiographic treatment response to dabrafenib and trametinib have been reported in a limited number of patients with BRAF-mutated PDAC who were nonresponsive to multiple lines of systemic therapy, but these responses were short-lived.[66]

From a precision therapeutics perspective, the necessity to identify fusion genes further highlights the importance of introducing NGS into clinical practice. This represents an urgent need, at least for patients with *KRAS* WT PDAC.

Promising Approaches

Compared to other cancers, precision medicine approaches are in their relative infancy for PDAC. Nonetheless, recent years have seen a rapid expansion of multiple initiatives taking place globally, with encouraging experiences showing the feasibility and clinical benefit of precision medicine-based approaches.

The feasibility of performing high-quality genomic profiling in clinically relevant timelines (<35 days) and identification of potentially actionable somatic as well as germline alterations in 48% of 71 patients analyzed (DDR gene mutations, *KRAS* WT tumors, *BRAF* alterations, and *ROS1* translocation) was recently demonstrated by Aguirre at al.[66] Data from the KYT initiative demonstrated the feasibility of screening patients with PDAC in a community setting and allocating them to a matched targeted therapy.[34,65] Of 1856 patients with PDAC referred to the KYT registry, 1082 patients (58%) received a molecular profiling report, which included actionable genomic alterations in 282 cases (26%). A retrospective analysis of patients for whom clinical follow-up was available showed that patients who received therapy matched to their genomic alterations ($n = 46$) had a significantly longer mOS time compared with those who received unmatched therapies ($n = 143$; 2.58 vs 1.51 years) or compared with those who did not possess an actionable molecular alteration (2.58 years vs 1.32 years). Notably, most of the patients who received matched therapy had predictive alterations in DDR genes.

Similarly, the COMPASS study demonstrated the feasibility of real-time WGS and RNA sequencing of advanced PC and its utility in identifying predictive mutational and transcriptional features for better treatment selection.[67,68] The results of this study showed an overall response rate of 10% for basal-like and of 33% for classic PDACs ($P = .02$). In patients treated with m-FOLFIRINOX, the progression rate was 60% in basal-like tumors compared with 15% in classic PDAC ($P = .0002$), with mOS of 5.9 months and 9.3 months for basal-like and classic, respectively (HR 0.47; 95% CI, 0.32–0.69, $P = .0001$). The findings of this trial proposed GATA6 as a surrogate biomarker for the differentiation between basal-like and classic subtypes but this finding needs further prospective validation.[68] In addition, potentially actionable genetic alterations were found in approximately 30% of patients, including *BRAF* (2%), *CDK4/6* (7%), *PIK3CA* (7%), *PTEN* (5%), and *RNF43* (3%) mutations.

Altogether, these studies demonstrated that a genomics-driven precision medicine strategy can be safely integrated into current clinical management with rapid turnaround time and has a high potential to drive both current and novel investigational therapeutic choices. However, only a small number of patients receive molecularly matched treatment, and major efforts are needed to conduct biomarker-directed clinical trials that are adequately powered for small subsets of patients carrying a diverse range of potentially actionable genetic aberrations.

Precision Medicine Approach to PDAC in 2021

To overcome the challenges of identifying low frequency of molecular alterations of interest, novel approaches using adaptive statistical designs and a master protocol to assign patients to different candidate drugs have shown promise in many tumor types. In this context, multiple platforms for therapeutic development are ongoing for PDAC, including the Precision Promise (NCT04229004), the PASS-01 (NCT04469556), and the Precision-Panc trials. The Precision-Panc trial aims to improve patient outcomes through the rapid translation of preclinical advances into a diverse range of PRIMUS (Pancreatic canceR Individualised Multi-arm Umbrella Study) trials, thus integrating the pivotal components of developmental therapeutics into the trial platform.

The tremendous intertumoral and intratumoral heterogeneity seen in PDAC combined with the robust contribution of the TME to defining tumor biology and therapeutic response necessitates the need to move away from standard histopathological classifications to a clinically relevant molecular taxonomy for all patients at the moment of initial diagnosis. Although this article focused on precision therapeutic approaches in PDAC, specifically aimed at the epithelial component of the tumor, there are several important efforts underway to target equally relevant components of the TME such as the stroma, the immune landscape, and distinct patterns of metabolism. Our evolving understanding of the complex pathophysiology of this disease will likely reveal the optimal precision therapeutic approach to PDAC treatment over the next decade.

OPPORTUNITIES AND CHALLENGES

Robust and concerted attempts at molecular classification of PDACs have yielded a wealth of data; however, a chasm exists between such data and routine clinical practice that needs to be bridged rapidly. There are several hurdles that need to be overcome: (i) the prognostic and to some extent predictive utility of the various classification schemes have been established, but the "OMIC" platform of choice for translation into clinical practice remains unclear; (ii) limited availability of tumor material for "OMICS"—in regular clinical practice, clinicians make treatment decisions based on limited tumor material available from endoscopic ultrasound–guided fine needle aspiration samples (in the neoadjuvant setting) or core biopsies in the metastatic setting; (iii) cost—the cost involved in such analysis may not currently be justified by

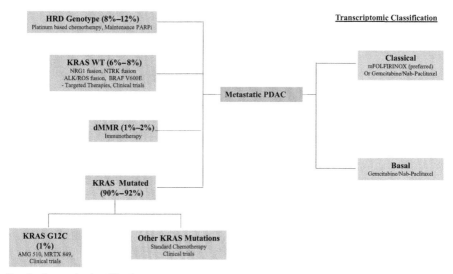

Fig. 1. Genomic classification.

the limited treatment options available and the existing insurance reimbursement model; (iv) lack of robust clinical decision support and bioinformatic tools to reliably and effectively reconcile "OMIC" data into clinically actionable "capsules" for the practicing clinician; and (v) pragmatic barriers to expedited "OMIC" profiling/reporting, identification of actionable biomarkers and enrollment in "personalized medicine" PDAC trials.[69–75]

Significant technologic and bioinformatic advances that have been realized over the past decade provide a glimpse of the substantial promise of precision medicine in the treatment of PDAC (**Fig. 1**). Specifically, identification of (i) substantial minority of patients with alterations in DDR genes and their likelihood of response to platinum/PARP therapy; (ii) *KRAS* WT patients with actionable somatic alterations; and (iii) predictive "OMIC" profiles using machine learning algorithms have immediate relevance in the therapeutic landscape of PDAC. Further refinement of the myriad "OMIC" strategies that are in various stages of development will likely transform the early detection, screening, diagnostic, and therapeutic options for this aggressive disease.

CLINICS CARE POINTS

- Germline testing should be performed for all patients with PDAC
- Somatic genomic profiling should be performed for all patients with advanced PDAC
- Germline alterations in DNA damage repair genes currently constitute the most prevalent actionable therapeutic target in pancreas cancer
- Germline and somatic mismatch repair deficiency status as well as various somatic fusion kinases serve as predictive biomarkers in a small subset of patients with pancreas cancer

DISCLOSURE

Consultant for Celgene, Ipsen, Foundation Medicine, Bristol-Myers Squibb, Exelixis, Taiho Oncology, and Roche/Genentech.

Research funding from Celgene, Foundation Medicine, Roche/Genentech, Boehringer Ingelheim, Tolero, Toray, Mirati, and NGM Biopharmaceuticals.

REFERENCES

1. Siegel RL, Miller KD, Fuchs HE, et al. Cancer Statistics, 2021. CA Cancer J Clin 2021;71(1):7–33.
2. Hruban RH, Goggins M, Parsons J, et al. Progression model for pancreatic cancer. Clin Cancer Res 2000;6(8):2969–72.
3. Lüttges J, Galehdari H, Bröcker V, et al. Allelic loss is often the first hit in the biallelic inactivation of the p53 and DPC4 genes during pancreatic carcinogenesis. Am J Pathol 2001;158(5):1677–83.
4. Moskaluk CA, Hruban RH, Kern SE. p16 and K-ras gene mutations in the intraductal precursors of human pancreatic adenocarcinoma. Cancer Res 1997; 57(11):2140–3.
5. Wilentz RE, Geradts J, Maynard R, et al. Inactivation of the p16 (INK4A) tumor-suppressor gene in pancreatic duct lesions: loss of intranuclear expression. Cancer Res 1998;58(20):4740–4.
6. Wilentz RE, Iacobuzio-Donahue CA, Argani P, et al. Loss of expression of Dpc4 in pancreatic intraepithelial neoplasia: evidence that DPC4 inactivation occurs late in neoplastic progression. Cancer Res 2000;60(7):2002–6.
7. Chari ST, Kelly K, Hollingsworth MA, et al. Early detection of sporadic pancreatic cancer: summative review. Pancreas 2015;44(5):693–712.
8. Cooper CS, Eeles R, Wedge DC, et al. Analysis of the genetic phylogeny of multifocal prostate cancer identifies multiple independent clonal expansions in neoplastic and morphologically normal prostate tissue. Nat Genet 2015;47(4): 367–72.
9. Martincorena I, Roshan A, Gerstung M, et al. Tumor evolution. High burden and pervasive positive selection of somatic mutations in normal human skin. Science 2015;348(6237):880–6.
10. Ross-Innes CS, Becq J, Warren A, et al. Whole-genome sequencing provides new insights into the clonal architecture of Barrett's esophagus and esophageal adenocarcinoma. Nat Genet 2015;47(9):1038–46.
11. Notta F, Chan-Seng-Yue M, Lemire M, et al. A renewed model of pancreatic cancer evolution based on genomic rearrangement patterns. Nature 2016; 538(7625):378–82.
12. Matthaei H, Schulick RD, Hruban RH, et al. Cystic precursors to invasive pancreatic cancer. Nat Rev Gastroenterol Hepatol 2011;8(3):141–50.
13. Winter JM, Cameron JL, Campbell KA, et al. 1423 pancreaticoduodenectomies for pancreatic cancer: A single-institution experience. J Gastrointest Surg 2006; 10(9):1199–210, discussion 1210-1.
14. Hahn SA, Greenhalf B, Ellis I, et al. BRCA2 germline mutations in familial pancreatic carcinoma. J Natl Cancer Inst 2003;95(3):214–21.
15. Jones S, Hruban RH, Kamiyama M, et al. Exomic sequencing identifies PALB2 as a pancreatic cancer susceptibility gene. Science 2009;324(5924):217.
16. Klein AP, Brune KA, Petersen GM, et al. Prospective risk of pancreatic cancer in familial pancreatic cancer kindreds. Cancer Res 2004;64(7):2634–8.

17. Rogers CD, van der Heijden MS, Brune K, et al. The genetics of FANCC and FANCG in familial pancreatic cancer. Cancer Biol Ther 2004;3(2):167–9.

18. Bardeesy N, Aguirre AJ, Chu GC, et al. Both p16(Ink4a) and the p19(Arf)-p53 pathway constrain progression of pancreatic adenocarcinoma in the mouse. Proc Natl Acad Sci U S A 2006;103(15):5947–52.

19. Hingorani SR, Wang L, Multani AS, et al. Trp53R172H and KrasG12D cooperate to promote chromosomal instability and widely metastatic pancreatic ductal adenocarcinoma in mice. Cancer Cell 2005;7(5):469–83.

20. Skoulidis F, Cassidy LD, Pisupati V, et al. Germline Brca2 heterozygosity promotes Kras(G12D) -driven carcinogenesis in a murine model of familial pancreatic cancer. Cancer Cell 2010;18(5):499–509.

21. Bailey P, Chang DK, Nones K, et al. Genomic analyses identify molecular subtypes of pancreatic cancer. Nature 2016;531(7592):47–52.

22. Biankin AV, Waddell N, Kassahn KS, et al. Pancreatic cancer genomes reveal aberrations in axon guidance pathway genes. Nature 2012;491(7424):399–405.

23. Jones S, Zhang X, Parsons DW, et al. Core signaling pathways in human pancreatic cancers revealed by global genomic analyses. Science 2008;321(5897): 1801–6.

24. Waddell N, Pajic M, Patch A-N, et al. Whole genomes redefine the mutational landscape of pancreatic cancer. Nature 2015;518(7540):495–501.

25. Collisson EA, Sadanandam A, Olson P, et al. Subtypes of pancreatic ductal adenocarcinoma and their differing responses to therapy. Nat Med 2011;17(4): 500–3.

26. Moffitt RA, Marayati R, Flate EL, et al. Virtual microdissection identifies distinct tumor- and stroma-specific subtypes of pancreatic ductal adenocarcinoma. Nat Genet 2015;47(10):1168–78.

27. Negrini S, Gorgoulis VG, Halazonetis TD. Genomic instability–an evolving hallmark of cancer. Nat Rev Mol Cell Biol 2010;11(3):220–8.

28. Grant RC, Selander I, Connor AA, et al. Prevalence of germline mutations in cancer predisposition genes in patients with pancreatic cancer. Gastroenterology 2015;148(3):556–64.

29. Hu C, Hart SN, Polley EC, et al. Association Between Inherited Germline Mutations in Cancer Predisposition Genes and Risk of Pancreatic Cancer. J Am Med Assoc 2018;319(23):2401–9.

30. Shindo K, Yu J, Suenaga M, et al. Deleterious Germline Mutations in Patients With Apparently Sporadic Pancreatic Adenocarcinoma. J Clin Oncol 2017;35(30): 3382–90.

31. Yurgelun MB, Chittenden AB, Morales-Oyarvide V, et al. Germline cancer susceptibility gene variants, somatic second hits, and survival outcomes in patients with resected pancreatic cancer. Genet Med 2019;21(1):213–23.

32. Jonsson P, Bandlamudi C, Cheng ML, et al. Tumour lineage shapes BRCA-mediated phenotypes. Nature 2019;571(7766):576–9.

33. Johnstone TC, Park GY, Lippard SJ. Understanding and improving platinum anticancer drugs–phenanthriplatin. Anticancer Res 2014;34(1):471–6.

34. Pishvaian MJ, Bender RJ, Halverson D, et al. Molecular Profiling of Patients with Pancreatic Cancer: Initial Results from the Know Your Tumor Initiative. Clin Cancer Res 2018;24(20):5018–27.

35. Wattenberg MM, Asch D, Yu S, et al. Platinum response characteristics of patients with pancreatic ductal adenocarcinoma and a germline BRCA1, BRCA2 or PALB2 mutation. Br J Cancer 2020;122(3):333–9.

36. Palacio S, de Almeida JCB, de Campos ÉA, et al. DNA damage repair deficiency as a predictive biomarker for FOLFIRINOX efficacy in metastatic pancreatic cancer. J Gastrointest Oncol 2019;10(6):1133–9.

37. Sehdev A, Gbolahan O, Hancock BA, et al. Germline and Somatic DNA Damage Repair Gene Mutations and Overall Survival in Metastatic Pancreatic Adenocarcinoma Patients Treated with FOLFIRINOX. Clin Cancer Res 2018;24(24): 6204–11.

38. Kondo T, Kanai M, Kou T, et al. Association between homologous recombination repair gene mutations and response to oxaliplatin in pancreatic cancer. Oncotarget 2018;9(28):19817–25.

39. Golan T, Kanji ZS, Epelbaum R, et al. Overall survival and clinical characteristics of pancreatic cancer in BRCA mutation carriers. Br J Cancer 2014;111(6): 1132–8.

40. Pilié PG, Tang C, Mills GB, et al. State-of-the-art strategies for targeting the DNA damage response in cancer. Nat Rev Clin Oncol 2019;16(2):81–104.

41. Golan T, Hammel P, Reni M, et al. Maintenance Olaparib for Germline BRCA-Mutated Metastatic Pancreatic Cancer. N Engl J Med 2019;381(4):317–27.

42. O'Reilly EM, Lee JW, Zalupski M, et al. Randomized, Multicenter, Phase II Trial of Gemcitabine and Cisplatin With or Without Veliparib in Patients With Pancreas Adenocarcinoma and a Germline BRCA/PALB2 Mutation. J Clin Oncol 2020; 38(13):1378–88.

43. O'Reilly EM, Lee JW, Lowery MA, et al. Phase 1 trial evaluating cisplatin, gemcitabine, and veliparib in 2 patient cohorts: Germline BRCA mutation carriers and wild-type BRCA pancreatic ductal adenocarcinoma. Cancer 2018;124(7): 1374–82.

44. Shroff RT, Hendifar A, McWilliams RR, et al. Rucaparib Monotherapy in Patients With Pancreatic Cancer and a Known Deleterious BRCA Mutation. JCO Precis Oncol 2018;2018.

45. Lowery MA, Kelsen DP, Capanu M, et al. Phase II trial of veliparib in patients with previously treated BRCA-mutated pancreas ductal adenocarcinoma. Eur J Cancer 2018;89:19–26.

46. Kaufman B, Shapira-Frommer R, Schmutzler RK, et al. Olaparib monotherapy in patients with advanced cancer and a germline BRCA1/2 mutation. J Clin Oncol 2015;33(3):244–50.

47. Lower SS, McGurk MP, Clark AG, et al. Satellite DNA evolution: old ideas, new approaches. Curr Opin Genet Dev 2018;49:70–8.

48. Hu ZI, Shia J, Stadler ZK, et al. Evaluating Mismatch Repair Deficiency in Pancreatic Adenocarcinoma: Challenges and Recommendations. Clin Cancer Res 2018;24(6):1326–36.

49. Latham A, Srinivasan P, Kemel Y, et al. Microsatellite Instability Is Associated With the Presence of Lynch Syndrome Pan-Cancer. J Clin Oncol 2019;37(4):286–95.

50. Le DT, Durham JN, Smith KN, et al. Mismatch repair deficiency predicts response of solid tumors to PD-1 blockade. Science 2017;357(6349):409–13.

51. Yachida S, Jones S, Bozic I, et al. Distant metastasis occurs late during the genetic evolution of pancreatic cancer. Nature 2010;467(7319):1114–7.

52. Pylayeva-Gupta Y, Grabocka E, Bar-Sagi D. RAS oncogenes: weaving a tumorigenic web. Nat Rev Cancer 2011;11(11):761–74.

53. Singh RR, Goldberg J, Varghese AM, et al. Genomic profiling in pancreatic ductal adenocarcinoma and a pathway towards therapy individualization: A scoping review. Cancer Treat Rev 2019;75:27–38.

54. Hong DS, Fakih MG, Strickler JH, et al. KRAS(G12C) Inhibition with Sotorasib in Advanced Solid Tumors. N Engl J Med 2020;383(13):1207–17.

55. Hallin J, Engstrom LD, Hargis L, et al. The KRAS(G12C) Inhibitor MRTX849 Provides Insight toward Therapeutic Susceptibility of KRAS-Mutant Cancers in Mouse Models and Patients. Cancer Discov 2020;10(1):54–71.

56. Zhou L, Baba Y, Kitano Y, et al. KRAS, BRAF, and PIK3CA mutations, and patient prognosis in 126 pancreatic cancers: pyrosequencing technology and literature review. Med Oncol 2016;33(4):32.

57. Heining C, Horak P, Uhrig S, et al. NRG1 Fusions in KRAS Wild-Type Pancreatic Cancer. Cancer Discov 2018;8(9):1087–95.

58. Singhi AD, George B, Greenbowe JR, et al. Real-Time Targeted Genome Profile Analysis of Pancreatic Ductal Adenocarcinomas Identifies Genetic Alterations That Might Be Targeted With Existing Drugs or Used as Biomarkers. Gastroenterology 2019;156(8):2242–53.e4.

59. Boeck S, Jung A, Laubender RP, et al. EGFR pathway biomarkers in erlotinib-treated patients with advanced pancreatic cancer: translational results from the randomised, crossover phase 3 trial AIO-PK0104. Br J Cancer 2013;108(2):469–76.

60. Nevala-Plagemann C, Hidalgo M, Garrido-Laguna I. From state-of-the-art treatments to novel therapies for advanced-stage pancreatic cancer. Nat Rev Clin Oncol 2020;17(2):108–23.

61. Drilon A, Laetsch TW, Kummar S, et al. Efficacy of Larotrectinib in TRK Fusion-Positive Cancers in Adults and Children. N Engl J Med 2018;378(8):731–9.

62. O'Reilly EM, Hechtman JF. Tumour response to TRK inhibition in a patient with pancreatic adenocarcinoma harbouring an NTRK gene fusion. Ann Oncol 2019;30(Suppl_8):viii36–40.

63. Foster SA, Whalen DM, Özen A, et al. Activation Mechanism of Oncogenic Deletion Mutations in BRAF, EGFR, and HER2. Cancer Cell 2016;29(4):477–93.

64. Lowery MA, Jordan EJ, Basturk O, et al. Real-Time Genomic Profiling of Pancreatic Ductal Adenocarcinoma: Potential Actionability and Correlation with Clinical Phenotype. Clin Cancer Res 2017;23(20):6094–100.

65. Pishvaian MJ, Blais EM, Brody JR, et al. Overall survival in patients with pancreatic cancer receiving matched therapies following molecular profiling: a retrospective analysis of the Know Your Tumor registry trial. Lancet Oncol 2020;21(4):508–18.

66. Aguirre AJ, Nowak JA, Camarda ND, et al. Real-time Genomic Characterization of Advanced Pancreatic Cancer to Enable Precision Medicine. Cancer Discov 2018;8(9):1096–111.

67. Aung KL, Fischer SE, Denroche RE, et al. Genomics-Driven Precision Medicine for Advanced Pancreatic Cancer: Early Results from the COMPASS Trial. Clin Cancer Res 2018;24(6):1344–54.

68. O'Kane GM, Grünwald BT, Jang GH, et al. GATA6 Expression Distinguishes Classical and Basal-like Subtypes in Advanced Pancreatic Cancer. Clin Cancer Res 2020;26(18):4901–10.

69. Chantrill LA, Nagrial AM, Watson C, et al. Precision Medicine for Advanced Pancreas Cancer: The Individualized Molecular Pancreatic Cancer Therapy (IMPaCT) Trial. Clin Cancer Res 2015;21(9):2029–37.

70. Kim ES, Herbst RS, Wistuba II, et al. The BATTLE trial: personalizing therapy for lung cancer. Cancer Discov 2011;1(1):44–53.

71. Le Tourneau C, Kamal M, Trédan O, et al. Designs and challenges for personalized medicine studies in oncology: focus on the SHIVA trial. Target Oncol 2012; 7(4):253–65.

72. Thompson AM, Jordan LB, Quinlan P, et al. Prospective comparison of switches in biomarker status between primary and recurrent breast cancer: the Breast Recurrence In Tissues Study (BRITS). Breast Cancer Res 2010;12(6):R92.

73. Tran B, Dancey JE, Kamel-Reid S, et al. Cancer genomics: technology, discovery, and translation. J Clin Oncol 2012;30(6):647–60.

74. Tsimberidou AM, Ringborg U, Schilsky RL. Strategies to overcome clinical, regulatory, and financial challenges in the implementation of personalized medicine. Am Soc Clin Oncol Educ Book 2013;118–25.

75. Von Hoff DD, Stephenson JJ Jr, Rosen P, et al. Pilot study using molecular profiling of patients' tumors to find potential targets and select treatments for their refractory cancers. J Clin Oncol 2010;28(33):4877–83.

Therapeutic Targeting of Autophagy in Pancreatic Cancer

Mona Foth, PhD[a], Ignacio Garrido-Laguna, MD, PhD[a,b], Conan G. Kinsey, MD, PhD[a,b,*]

KEYWORDS

- Pancreatic cancer • Autophagy • Therapeutics • Pancreatic cancer clinical trials
- Autophagy clinical trials

KEY POINTS

- Inhibiting autophagy may be a therapeutic opportunity in pancreatic cancer.
- Clinical trials using hydroxychloroquine for autophagy inhibition have, as of yet, not demonstrated mPFS or mOS efficacy in patients with pancreatic cancer
- Combining autophagy inhibition with targeted and/or immunotherapy may be efficacious with many clinical trials ongoing.
- Several chloroquine chemical derivatives and more specific autophagy inhibitors are in preclinical and clinical development.

INTRODUCTION

Macroautophagy (herein referred to as autophagy) is an evolutionarily conserved process by which intracellular macromolecules and organelles are degraded to recycle biosynthetic substrates for further cellular growth and metabolism by packaging cytosolic components, including organelles, into vesicles (autophagosomes), which are then fused with lysosomes (**Fig. 1**). These autolysosomes lead to the subsequent degradation of the internal components and release of metabolites for further cell metabolism and proliferation. In cancer biology the role of autophagy is complex and how it affects malignant cell function is only partially understood. In pancreatic ductal adenocarcinoma (PDAC) autophagy upregulation has been shown in several PDAC cell lines, as well as incremental autophagy upregulation in the progression of normal pancreatic tissue to pancreatic intraductal neoplasia (PanIN) to PDAC,[1,2] suggesting a protumorigenic role.

[a] Huntsman Cancer Institute, University of Utah, 2000 Circle of Hope, Salt Lake City, UT 84112, USA; [b] Department of Internal Medicine, Division of Oncology, University of Utah School of Medicine, 30 North 1900 East, Salt Lake City, UT 84132, USA
* Corresponding author.
E-mail address: Conan.Kinsey@hci.utah.edu
Twitter: @ConanKinsey (C.G.K.)

Surg Oncol Clin N Am 30 (2021) 709–718
https://doi.org/10.1016/j.soc.2021.06.001
1055-3207/21/Published by Elsevier Inc.

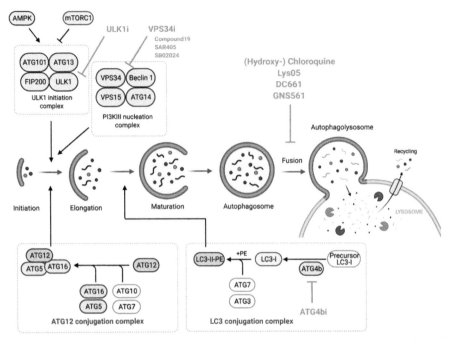

Fig. 1. Overview of autophagy and pharmacologic inhibitors. Autophagy is used by the cell to package cytosolic components and organelles into vesicles for degradation and recycling. ULK1 (ATG1), the "master regulator" of autophagy is activated by the AMPK signaling pathway and inactivated by the mTORC1 signaling pathway. ULK1 then complexes with other autophagy machinery proteins into an ULK1 initiation complex, which then partners with the VPS34 complex and the ATG12 conjugation complex to initiate membrane formation of the autophagosome vesicle. The forming autophagosome is then tagged with LC3-II by the LC3 conjugation complex, and LC3-II acts as a scaffold protein for other cellular machinery to traffic the autophagosome within the cytoplasm, and for eventual fusion with lysosomes. Once fused with lysosomes the fused vesicle is now an autophagolysosome wherein the cargo and inner membrane are degraded releasing biosynthetic substrates for further cellular growth and metabolism. Various inhibitory steps and compounds are listed in green.

To address whether autophagy is required for PDAC tumor progression and maintenance, Yang and colleagues[3] used a genetically engineered mouse model of PDAC *(Pdx1^{Cre+}, LSL-Kras$^{G12D/+}$, Trp53$^{lox/+}$)* with either heterozygous or homozygous deletion of the essential autophagy gene *Atg5*. The loss of *Atg5* in tumor cells resulted in the expected autophagy inhibition and increased PanINs, but less progression to PDAC. Furthermore, treatment with the autophagy inhibitors chloroquine or hydroxychloroquine of murine PDAC cell lines and patient-derived PDAC xenografts led to increased apoptosis and decreased proliferation.

Further studies used a genetically engineered mouse model of PDAC (*LSL-Kras^{G12D}, Trp53$^{lox/+}$, p48^{Cre+}*) expressing a doxycycline-inducible dominant negative *Atg4b* (*Atg4b^{C74A}*).[4] ATG4B is required for autophagosome formation, and the addition of doxycycline to mouse diet results in the expression of dominant negative Atg4b and subsequent autophagy inhibition, which can be reversed by removing doxycycline from the diet. The investigators demonstrated that strong autophagy inhibition by expression of dominant negative Atg4b from 2 alleles in established PDAC tumors resulted in complete tumor regression. Furthermore, in mice that were heterozygous for the dominant negative *Atg4b*, the mutant allele was lost and autophagy restored in PDAC tumors that continued to grow, suggesting a dependence on autophagy for PDAC tumor proliferation. Previous studies had demonstrated a possible tumor suppressive role for autophagy, which would have negative implications in using autophagy inhibition as a therapeutic strategy.[5-7] Although with continuous autophagy inhibition in the presence of mutant KRAS there was extensive pancreatic metaplasia, without mutant KRAS no metaplasia or tumors were observed. It was also demonstrated that intermittent autophagy inhibition did not induce metaplasia even in the KRAS mutant background. This suggested that mutant KRAS was required for continuous autophagy inhibition to induce metaplasia and that autophagy inhibition in normal tissue would not result in progression to malignant transformation. These studies indicated that autophagy was essential for PDAC tumor growth and maintenance and that targeting autophagy might be a viable therapeutic strategy.

Hydroxychloroquine to Inhibit Autophagy for Metastatic Pancreatic Ductal Adenocarcinoma

The antimalarial 4-aminoquinolines chloroquine and hydroxychloroquine have been well documented to inhibit autophagy. This inhibition was believed to be due to alkylinization of the lysosomal compartment, which typically requires an acidic environment for enzymatic degradation within the lysosome; however, more recent data have indicated that the protein palmitoyl-protein thioesterase 1 (PPT1) may be the target of chloroquine and hydroxychloroquine.[8,9] Indeed, many of the side effects of chloroquine and hydroxychloroquine, such as retinopathy and vision loss, are recapitulated by loss of PPT1 function in humans. Given that 4-aminoquinolines have been approved by the US Food and Drug Administration (FDA) for the past 70 years and are still used off-label for the treatment of rheumatoid arthritis and lupus erythematosus, these compounds were easily repurposed for the studies of the treatment of PDAC.

Hydroxychloroquine was studied as a single-agent therapy in a phase II trial for metastatic PDAC in the third-line setting in patients who were Eastern Cooperative Oncology Group (ECOG) grade 0 to 2. Ten patients were administered 400 mg twice daily and 10 patients were administered 600 mg twice daily (maximum dose approved by the FDA)[10]; 10% of patients were without progressive disease at 2 months. With a median progression-free survival (mPFS) and median overall survival (mOS) of 46.5 and 69.0 days, respectively, it was determined that single-agent hydroxychloroquine lacked efficacy in this patient population. It should be noted, however, that the study used biochemical markers from peripheral lymphocytes to identify if autophagy was indeed inhibited and found inconsistent results.

Preclinical data demonstrated that autophagy inhibition with chloroquine/hydroxychloroquine may enhance the efficacy of chemotherapy.[11] A phase II trial examined combining hydroxychloroquine with gemcitabine/nab-paclitaxel with a 1:1 enrollment to receive gemcitabine/nab-paclitaxel at standard dosing with or without hydroxychloroquine 600 mg by mouth twice daily in 112 patients with untreated metastatic or advanced, unresectable disease who were ECOG grade 0 to 1 (NCT01506973).[12] The primary objective was mOS at 1 year, which was 41% for the gemcitabine/nab-paclitaxel/hydroxychloroquine group and 49% for the gemcitabine/nab-paclitaxel group. These data did not support the addition of hydroxychloroquine to gemcitabine/nab-paclitaxel. However, the addition of hydroxychloroquine did show a statistically significant improvement in overall response rate (ORR) from 21% to 38%. Although encouraging, this ORR could have been overestimated given the small study size.

As a single agent or in combination with chemotherapy hydroxychloroquine had no efficacy in improving mOS for patients with metastatic PDAC. This lack of efficacy could be potentially due to inefficacy as a single agent or in combination with chemotherapy or the weak autophagy inhibitory effect of hydroxychloroquine at the maximum dose allowed by the FDA. At present, there are 2 ongoing trials, one combining gemcitabine and nab-paclitaxel with hydroxychloroquine and paricalcitol for advanced or metastatic PDAC and one combining gemcitabine, nab-paclitaxel, cisplatin, and hydroxychloroquine for untreated pancreatic cancer; however, the results have not been reported yet (NCT04524702 and NCT04669197). Although efficacy was not demonstrated for mOS, the modest possible improvement in ORR seen in combination with chemotherapy was an initiative to investigate whether hydroxychloroquine could have some therapeutic benefit in the neoadjuvant setting.

Hydroxychloroquine with Chemotherapy for Neoadjuvant Pancreatic Ductal Adenocarcinoma Treatment

Given the aforementioned phase II trial data demonstrating a statistically significant ORR improvement with the addition of hydroxychloroquine to standard-of-care chemotherapy, 2 studies sought to investigate the possible benefit of autophagy inhibition in the neoadjuvant setting for PDAC.

One study was a single-arm phase II study that added hydroxychloroquine to neoadjuvant chemoradiation in patients with potentially resectable PDAC (NCT01494155).[13] The primary outcome was mPFS with secondary outcomes including pathologic response rate and mOS. Hydroxychloroquine was started 1 week before starting chemoradiation and continued until the day before surgery. For standard-of-care treatment patients received either 5 Gy × 5 with protons or 3 Gy × 10 with photons concurrent with capecitabine 825 mg/m^2 twice daily for weeks 1 and 2 Monday through Friday. Surgery was then performed 1 to 3 weeks postcompletion of chemoradiation. After surgical recovery patients went on to restart hydroxychloroquine and also receive 6 months of gemcitabine-based adjuvant chemotherapy. Patients continued hydroxychloroquine until progression. Of the 50 patients who were enrolled in the study 47 went on to resection; 38 patients had an R0 resection and 9 patients had an R1 resection, and 31 of 47 patients had positive lymph nodes. mPFS was 12 months and mOS was 18.7 months. Three patients in the study had grade 3 toxicities (6%). It was concluded that although the regimen was well tolerated, there was no meaningful impact on mOS.

The other study was a randomized phase II study that tested nab-paclitaxel and gemcitabine (PG) versus nab-paclitaxel, gemcitabine, and hydroxychloroquine (PGH) in patients with potentially resectable PDAC (NCT01978184).[14] The primary end point was histopathologic response in the resected specimen. Secondary clinical end points included serum CA 19-9 biomarker response, and exploratory end points included markers of autophagy. In this study 52 patients were randomized to the PGH arm and 46 patients to the PG arm, and 34 and 30 patients were evaluable for the primary end point for the PGH and PG arms, respectively. There were no differences in serious adverse advents between the treatment groups. The PGH arm demonstrated statistically significant improvement in Evans grade histopathologic scores compared with the PG arm. There were 19 patients in the PGH arm who had an Evans IIB grade (>50% destruction of tumor cells) or greater response, versus 3 participants in the PG arm (55.9% vs 10%). No patients in the PG arm had an Evans grade III response (>90% destruction) versus 7 patients in the PGH arm (20.6%). Overall, Evans grade histopathologic response was statistically significant between the 2 arms in favor of PGH (Fisher exact test, $P = .004$). In addition, there was a statistically significant improvement of CA19-9 posttreatment to pretreatment ratios. Interestingly, the PGH group also had less lymph node involvement at the time of surgery, 58.8% versus 80%, but this was not statistically significant. Although the pathologic and biochemical response rates seem to favor adding hydroxychloroquine to neoadjuvant chemotherapy, the mOS and relapse-free survival did not differ between the groups.

Both of these studies tested whether autophagy inhibition by hydroxychloroquine could improve outcomes for patients in the neoadjuvant setting. Although one study did show improved pathologic and biochemical responses that were statistically significant by adding hydroxychloroquine to neoadjuvant chemotherapy, this did not translate to improvement in overall survival or relapse-free survival. Further studies adding hydroxychloroquine to FOLFIRINOX in the neoadjuvant setting have been suggested, but have yet to be implemented.

Combining Hydroxychloroquine with Targeted Therapies

More recently it was discovered that inhibition of the RAS-RAF-MEK-ERK MAPK kinase pathway results in the induction of autophagy. Autophagy induction was first observed in *BRAF*-mutated malignancies with BRAF inhibition.[15–18] Combining BRAF inhibition with hydroxychloroquine demonstrated possible efficacy in overcoming resistance in pediatric brain tumors to BRAF inhibition, as well as extending progression-free survival in *BRAF*-mutated melanoma with BRAF/MEK inhibition plus hydroxychloroquine (NCT02257424).

Further studies identified the induction of autophagy in *RAS*-mutated malignancies with MEK or ERK inhibition, and combined treatment of preclinical models with hydroxychloroquine resulted in synergistic tumor regression and suppression, whereas single agents had little effect, most notably in PDAC.[19,20] Furthermore, off-label treatment of a single patient with metastatic PDAC resulted in an impressive 50% reduction in tumor burden after the patient had demonstrated resistance to 3 prior lines of chemotherapy. This was remarkable given that MEK inhibition and hydroxychloroquine were both shown to be ineffective either in combination with chemotherapy or as single agents.[10,21] Further case reports have demonstrated stabilization of PDAC in 2 other patients with metastatic PDAC.[22] Several phase I clinical trials are ongoing to test the safety and tolerability of combining MEK1/2 or ERK1/2 inhibition and hydroxychloroquine (NCT04132505, NCT03825289, NCT04386057, NCT04145297) in PDAC.

In addition, other targeted therapies have been observed to induce autophagy in PDAC. Ji and colleagues[23] demonstrated that CDK4/6 inhibition with palbociclib resulted in induction of autophagy, which could be blocked with hydroxychloroquine. Similar to the combination of ERK or MEK inhibition with chloroquine/hydroxychloroquine, the combination of palbociclib and hydroxychloroquine resulted in a synergistic antiproliferative effect on PDAC cell lines.

These data suggest that various targeted therapies result in autophagy induction, likely as a protective mechanism, and blockade of this protective autophagy results in synergistic antiproliferation and apoptosis in PDAC cells. Identification of other possible targeted therapy combinations with autophagy inhibition are likely to occur in the near future.

Combining Hydroxychloroquine with Immunotherapy

The promise of immunotherapy has been successfully implemented in many other forms of cancer; however, PDAC remains a recalcitrant target for this new treatment modality; this may, in part, be due to the high levels of autophagic activity within PDAC cells. Yamamoto and colleagues[24] recently demonstrated that blockade of autophagy resulted in increased major histocompatibility complex (MHC)-1 expression on the cell surface of PDAC cells. It was determined that MHC-1 molecules were selectively targeted to autophagosomes and then subsequently degraded. Inhibition of autophagy restored MHC-I molecules to the cell surface, and treatment of orthotopic, syngeneic PDAC tumors with chloroquine, anti-PD-1, and anti-CTLA4 resulted in tumor regression, whereas treatment with chloroquine or anti-PD-1, and anti-CTLA had no effect.

Furthermore, Jiang and colleagues[25] tested the combination of trametinib; mefloquine, a 4-aminoquinolone similar to chloroquine/hydroxychloroquine; and CD40 agonist in an orthotopic, syngeneic mouse model of PDAC. The investigators demonstrated that the triple combination of MEK inhibition, autophagy inhibition, and immunotherapy with CD40 agonist resulted in tumor regression, some apparent cures, and extension of overall survival. Furthermore, mice that were cured were reimplanted with PDAC cells without engraftment, suggesting a robust immune response against the PDAC cells.

At present, there is a clinical trial investigating the combination of autophagy inhibition with immunotherapy in combination with MEK inhibition in PDAC (NCT04214418). The MEKiAUTO trial combines cobimetinib, atezolizumab, and hydroxychloroquine in patients with PDAC and is currently in phase I with plan to expand to phase II. Given the aforementioned data it is likely that we will see more clinical trials combining autophagy inhibitors with immunotherapeutic agents in the near future.

New Therapeutic Agents Targeting Autophagy

To date, all clinical trials investigating autophagy inhibition have used chloroquine or hydroxychloroquine because of prior FDA approval and a well-known toxicity profile; however, these compounds are pleotropic with many off-target effects involving other cellular processes requiring lysosomal function, as well as mitochondrial function. In addition, hydroxychloroquine and chloroquine are weak autophagy inhibitors requiring high concentrations resulting in increased frequency of off-target side effects. More specific and potent inhibitors of autophagy are currently under investigation and will undoubtedly be investigated in first-in-human clinical trials in the near future.

As chloroquine and hydroxychloroquine are weak inhibitors of autophagy and have a predefined maximum tolerable dose from the FDA, there has been interest in developing more potent analogues of 4-aminoquinolones. By essentially linking 2 chloroquine molecules, McAfee and colleagues[26] demonstrated a 10-fold increase in the potency to inhibit autophagy of the compound named Lys01 compared with chloroquine or hydroxychloroquine. Further chemical manipulations resulted in a compound named Lys05, which was more soluble in aqueous solution, but retained the 10-fold potency of Lys01.[26] PDAC xenografts treated with Lys05 demonstrated tumor growth suppression and stabilization, but no regressions. Building on the concept of dimerizing 4-aminoquinolines, Rebecca and colleagues[9] derived a compound named DC661, a dimeric chloroquine with a longer chemical linker than Lys05. This compound was reported to be 100-fold more potent than hydroxychloroquine, and treatment of colon cancer cell line-xenografted tumors resulted in complete suppression of tumor formation. Another 4-aminoquinoline derivative, GNS561, is currently in clinical trials for cholangiocarcinoma and hepatocellular carcinoma, but has yet to disclose results (NCT03316222). These compounds represent a possible alternative to chloroquine and hydroxychloroquine in clinical trials. However, although potentially more potent at inhibiting lysosomal function and therefore the final step in autophagy, the side effects exhibited by 4-aminoquinolines at higher doses, for example, irreversible retinopathy and vision loss, may also become more pronounced in the dimeric quinacrine compounds.

The protein VPS34 is a class III phosphoinositide 3-kinase (PI3K) that is involved in autophagosome formation by producing phosphatidylinositol-3-phosphate in the forming autophagosome membrane, which in turn acts as a binding site for further ATG proteins involved in autophagosome formation. As small-molecular-weight inhibitors for other PI3K enzymes have been developed, this is an attractive target for autophagy inhibition. Honda and colleagues demonstrated that a VPS34 inhibitor referred to as compound 19 resulted in both *in vitro* and *in vivo* autophagy inhibition in biochemical assays; however, human-derived colon cancer cell line xenografts failed to respond to single-agent treatment.[27] Furthermore, 2 other VPS34 inhibitor compounds, SAR405 and SB02024, did demonstrate tumor growth reduction, but not regression in mouse model-derived melanoma, colon cancer, and renal cell carcinoma cell lines.[28] Tumor growth reduction was potentiated by the addition of anti-PD-1/PD-L1 therapies to these VPS34 inhibitors, but frank tumor reductions were not observed.

ULK1 is a protein kinase that is phosphorylated by AMPK and mTORC1 resulting in activation and inhibition, respectively. Owing to it being the convergence point of 2 nutrient-sensing pathways and indispensable for canonical autophagy it has been deemed "the master regulator" of autophagy. Lazarus and colleagues[29] and Egan and colleagues[30] demonstrated that ATP competitive inhibitors could be developed for ULK1. Several ULK1 inhibitors are currently under development with some prepared to go into first-in-human clinical trials. Although this is an exciting development to have a first-in-class, specific autophagy inhibitor, there are noncanonical, ULK1-independent forms of autophagy that could potentially bypass ULK1 inhibition.[31] Whether PDAC will use these noncanonical autophagy pathways that do not depend on ULK1 to be primarily refractory or become resistant remains to be seen.

ATG4B is a cysteine protease that is involved in the cleavage of pro-LC3 to LC3-I, which is subsequently conjugated to lipid membranes and acts as a scaffold for further autophagosome formation and vesicular trafficking within the cell. Given the previously described work by Yang and colleagues[4] ATG4B represents an attractive target for autophagy inhibition. As ATG4B is a cysteine protease, there is a potential to develop potent covalent inhibitors similar to the KRAS^{G12C} inhibitor AMG-510. Although preclinical studies have demonstrated effective autophagy inhibition with ATG4B inhibitory compounds and possible preclinical efficacy, first-in-human trials are still awaited.

Challenges and Future Directions

Although autophagy seems to be an attractive therapeutic target for PDAC many barriers to clinical study still remain. As previously mentioned, the only autophagy inhibitors that are currently available are chloroquine and hydroxychloroquine; however, many new and more targeted autophagy inhibitors are in development. Although targeting autophagy more specifically may be advantageous, it may also allow for resistance to arise more quickly as the PDAC cells adapt to supply their energy needs through other nutrient-acquiring mechanisms, such as engulfing macromolecules from the extracellular environment, for example, macropinocytosis.[32,33] Although lysosomal inhibitors, such as chloroquine and hydroxychloroquine, are more pleotropic, they also inhibit other pathways, such as macropinocytosis, that require lysosomal function for the final step of degradation. It may be that lysosomal inhibitors are more effective due to the more pleotropic effects on multiple nutrient-acquiring pathways; however, this will remain unknown until the more specific autophagy inhibitors are tested in a clinical setting.

Another challenge to studying autophagy inhibition is the lack of surrogate biomarkers for autophagy blockade. Autophagy inhibition in peripheral leukocytes and lymphocytes has been previously investigated as a surrogate biomarker with inconsistent results.[10] In addition, using peripheral blood cells is also a poor surrogate for autophagy activity within the tumor because drug concentrations may differ between the tumor microenvironment and the peripheral blood. p62 (SQSTM1), a protein that accumulates when autophagy is inhibited, was used as a biomarker for autophagy inhibition in clinical studies through immunohistochemistry for p62 on formalin-fixed, paraffin-embedded tumor samples.[14] A significant increase in p62-positive cells was observed in patients who were treated with hydroxychloroquine plus chemotherapy versus those treated with chemotherapy alone (43.6; 95% confidence interval [CI], 31.7–55.6 vs 27.5; 95% CI, 16.6–38.8; $P = .027$); this may be a viable biochemical surrogate for autophagy inhibition; however, it requires that tumor samples be obtained. Obtaining samples is not an issue for neoadjuvant trials, but can be difficult for adjuvant or palliative trials. Given that p62 accumulates when autophagy is inhibited, and tumor cells in which autophagy is inhibited are more likely to undergo apoptosis/necrosis resulting in cell lysis, there may be an opportunity to measure p62 protein levels in the bloodstream as a surrogate marker, however, this hypothesis remains to be tested.

Since Yoshinori Ohsumi's first experiments describing and dissecting the cellular process of autophagy in the early 1990s the field has rapidly advanced to a more complete, but still partial, understanding of this complex and integral part of cell biology. We have identified autophagy as aberrantly upregulated in many forms of cancer, including PDAC, and therefore a possible Achilles' heel to more specifically target cancer cells. Currently there are 173 trials that list autophagy as a target on clinicaltrials. gov, and this will only expand as we are on the cusp of having at our disposal an array of diverse, potent, and specific autophagy inhibitors to test clinically in the near future.

DISCLOSURE STATEMENT

Mona Foth: None to disclose.

Ignacio Garrido-Laguna: None to disclose.

Conan G. Kinsey: Dr Kinsey is a consultant for Deciphera Pharmaceuticals and SpringWorks Therapeutics.

REFERENCES

1. Yang S, Wang X, Contino G, et al. Pancreatic cancers require autophagy for tumor growth. Genes Dev 2011;25(7):717–29.

2. Kinsey C, Balakrishnan V, O'Dell MR, et al. Plac8 links oncogenic mutations to regulation of autophagy and is critical to pancreatic cancer progression. Cell Rep 2014;7(4):1143–55.

3. Yang A, Rajeshkumar NV, Wang X, et al. Autophagy is critical for pancreatic tumor growth and progression in tumors with p53 alterations. Cancer Discov 2014;4(8): 905–13.

4. Yang A, Herter-Sprie G, Zhang H, et al. Autophagy sustains pancreatic cancer growth through both cell-autonomous and nonautonomous mechanisms. Cancer Discov 2018;8(3):276–87.

5. Rosenfeldt MT, O'Prey J, Morton JP, et al. p53 status determines the role of autophagy in pancreatic tumour development. Nature 2013;504(7479):296–300.

6. Yue Z, Jin S, Yang C, Levine AJ, Heintz N. Beclin 1, an autophagy gene essential for early embryonic development, is a haploinsufficient tumor suppressor. Proc Natl Acad Sci U S A 2003;100(25):15077–82.

7. Qu X, Yu J, Bhagat G, et al. Promotion of tumorigenesis by heterozygous disruption of the beclin 1 autophagy gene. J Clin Invest 2003;112(12):1809–20.

8. Rebecca VW, Nicastri MC, McLaughlin N, et al. A unified approach to targeting the lysosome's degradative and growth signaling roles. Cancer Discov 2017; 7(11):1266–83.

9. Rebecca VW, Nicastri MC, Fennelly C, et al. PPT1 promotes tumor growth and is the molecular target of chloroquine derivatives in cancer. Cancer Discov 2019; 9(2):220–9.

10. Wolpin BM, Rubinson DA, Wang X, et al. Phase II and pharmacodynamic study of autophagy inhibition using hydroxychloroquine in patients with metastatic pancreatic adenocarcinoma. Oncologist 2014;19(6):637–8.

11. Amaravadi RK, Yu D, Lum JJ, et al. Autophagy inhibition enhances therapy-induced apoptosis in a Myc-induced model of lymphoma. J Clin Invest 2007; 117(2):326–36.

12. Karasic TB, O'Hara MH, Loaiza-Bonilla A, et al. Effect of gemcitabine and nab-paclitaxel with or without hydroxychloroquine on patients with advanced pancreatic cancer: a phase 2 randomized clinical trial. JAMA Oncol 2019;5(7):993–8.

13. Hong TS, Wo JY-L, Jiang W, et al. Phase II study of autophagy inhibition with hydroxychloroquine (HCQ) and preoperative (preop) short course chemoradiation (SCRT) followed by early surgery for resectable ductal adenocarcinoma of the head of pancreas (PDAC). J Clin Oncol 2017;35(15_suppl):4118.

14. Zeh HJ, Bahary N, Boone BA, et al. A randomized phase II preoperative study of autophagy inhibition with high-dose hydroxychloroquine and gemcitabine/Nab-paclitaxel in pancreatic cancer patients. Clin Cancer Res 2020;26(13):3126–34.

15. Levy JM, Thompson JC, Griesinger AM, et al. Autophagy inhibition improves chemosensitivity in BRAF(V600E) brain tumors. Cancer Discov 2014;4(7):773–80.

16. Wang W, Kang H, Zhao Y, et al. Targeting autophagy sensitizes BRAF-mutant thyroid cancer to vemurafenib. J Clin Endocrinol Metab 2017;102(2):634–43.

17. Ma XH, Piao SF, Dey S, et al. Targeting ER stress-induced autophagy overcomes BRAF inhibitor resistance in melanoma. J Clin Invest 2014;124(3):1406–17.

18. Li S, Song Y, Quach C, et al. Transcriptional regulation of autophagy-lysosomal function in BRAF-driven melanoma progression and chemoresistance. Nat Commun 2019;10(1):1693.

19. Bryant KL, Stalnecker CA, Zeitouni D, et al. Combination of ERK and autophagy inhibition as a treatment approach for pancreatic cancer. Nat Med 2019;25(4): 628–40.

20. Kinsey CG, Camolotto SA, Boespflug AM, et al. Protective autophagy elicited by RAF–>MEK–>ERK inhibition suggests a treatment strategy for RAS-driven cancers. Nat Med 2019;25(4):620–7.

21. Infante JR, Somer BG, Park JO, et al. A randomised, double-blind, placebo-controlled trial of trametinib, an oral MEK inhibitor, in combination with gemcitabine for patients with untreated metastatic adenocarcinoma of the pancreas. Eur J Cancer 2014;50(12):2072–81.

22. Xavier CB, Marchetti KR, Castria TB, Jardim DLF, Fernandes GS. Trametinib and Hydroxychloroquine (HCQ) combination treatment in KRAS-mutated advanced pancreatic adenocarcinoma: detailed description of two cases. J Gastrointest Cancer 2021;52(1):374–80.

23. Ji Y, Liu X, Li J, et al. Use of ratiometrically designed nanocarrier targeting CDK4/6 and autophagy pathways for effective pancreatic cancer treatment. Nat Commun 2020;11(1):4249.

24. Yamamoto K, Venida A, Yano J, et al. Autophagy promotes immune evasion of pancreatic cancer by degrading MHC-I. Nature 2020;581(7806):100–5.

25. Jiang H, Courau T, Lupin-Jimenez L, et al. Activating immune recognition in pancreatic ductal adenocarcinoma using autophagy inhibition, MEK blockade and CD40 agonism. bioRxiv 2020;2020. 2011.2005.370569.

26. McAfee Q, Zhang Z, Samanta A, et al. Autophagy inhibitor Lys05 has single-agent antitumor activity and reproduces the phenotype of a genetic autophagy deficiency. Proc Natl Acad Sci U S A 2012;109(21):8253–8.

27. Honda A, Harrington E, Cornella-Taracido I, et al. Potent, selective, and orally bioavailable inhibitors of VPS34 provide chemical tools to modulate autophagy in vivo. ACS Med Chem Lett 2016;7(1):72–6.

28. Noman MZ, Parpal S, Van Moer K, et al. Inhibition of Vps34 reprograms cold into hot inflamed tumors and improves anti-PD-1/PD-L1 immunotherapy. Sci Adv 2020;6(18):eaax7881.

29. Lazarus MB, Novotny CJ, Shokat KM. Structure of the human autophagy initiating kinase ULK1 in complex with potent inhibitors. ACS Chem Biol 2015;10(1):257–61.

30. Egan DF, Shackelford DB, Mihaylova MM, et al. Phosphorylation of ULK1 (hATG1) by AMP-activated protein kinase connects energy sensing to mitophagy. Science 2011;331(6016):456–61.

31. Cheong H, Lindsten T, Wu J, Lu C, Thompson CB. Ammonia-induced autophagy is independent of ULK1/ULK2 kinases. Proc Natl Acad Sci U S A 2011;108(27):11121–6.

32. Su H, Yang F, Fu R, et al. Cancer cells escape autophagy inhibition via NRF2-induced macropinocytosis. Cancer Cell 2021;39(5):678–93.e1.

33. Alers S, Loffler AS, Paasch F, et al. Atg13 and FIP200 act independently of Ulk1 and Ulk2 in autophagy induction. Autophagy 2011;7(12):1423–33.

Evolving Concepts Regarding Radiation Therapy for Pancreatic Cancer

William A. Hall, MD[a,b,c,*], Beth Erickson, MD[a,c],
Christopher H. Crane, MD[d]

KEYWORDS

- MR-guided radiation therapy • Pancreatic radiation dose escalation
- MR-guided RT for pancreatic cancer

KEY POINTS

- Local recurrence and progression both are common and morbid events in pancreatic cancer.
- Most historic neoadjuvant trials for pancreatic adenocarcinoma have included some type of radiation therapy.
- Radiation therapy is dramatically changing and deserves careful consideration by surgical oncologists for its potential benefits.

INTRODUCTION

Pancreatic ductal adenocarcinoma (PDAC) has one of the highest mortality to incidence rates of any solid tumor.[1] Local disease-related morbidity contributes significantly to the very poor overall survival (OS). Tragically, PDAC has higher rates of local recurrence and margin-positive resections than any other solid tumor managed with curative surgical resection. Compared with primary adenocarcinomas of the rectum, colon, lung, prostate, and breast, rates of margin positivity and local recurrence are magnitudes higher in PDAC.[2] Driven by this recurrence risk, radiation therapy (RT) has been an integral part of treatment strategies for PDAC for decades. Over this same period of time, the precise role of RT has become increasingly controversial. In today's practice, most institutions individualize the use of adjuvant, neoadjuvant,

---

[a] Department of Radiation Oncology, Froedtert and the Medical College of Wisconsin, 8701 West Watertown Plank Road, Milwaukee, WI 53226, USA; [b] Graduate School of Biomedical Sciences, Medical College of Wisconsin; [c] Department of Surgery, Froedtert and the Medical College of Wisconsin; [d] Department of Radiation Oncology, Memorial Sloan Kettering Cancer Center
* Corresponding author.
E-mail address: whall@mcw.edu
Twitter: @whallradonc (W.A.H.)

Surg Oncol Clin N Am 30 (2021) 719–730
https://doi.org/10.1016/j.soc.2021.06.009
1055-3207/21/© 2021 Elsevier Inc. All rights reserved.

and definitive RT based on their interpretation of the available data. This is due to the limitations of the interpretation of randomized data and the absence of well-powered clinical trials evaluating role of RT in this disease. This review highlights novel concepts and approaches to the use of RT that should be considered by the surgical oncologist.

UNIQUE ASPECTS OF RADIATION THERAPY COMPARED WITH CHEMOTHERAPY

Chemotherapy currently represents the backbone in managing of all stages of PDAC. Local recurrence, distant recurrence, and OS remain poor, however, even in the most modern trials.[3] For intact local tumors, the interstitial pressure in the stroma is thought to limit chemotherapy delivery to the primary tumor.[4] Thus far, there seems to be a limit to the survival duration that can be achieved with chemotherapy alone. Local treatments like surgery and ablative radiation, therefore, are critical in the optimal management in patients with localized disease.[5]

The only curative management strategy currently available in PDAC is multimodality therapy, consisting of surgical resection, chemotherapy, and in many circumstances RT. Unfortunately, only a small minority of patients are even eligible for surgery. Of those patients who undergo surgery, only a small percentage complete all intended therapy.[6–8] If a local modality could achieve similar local tumor control as surgical resection, curative treatment could be accomplished in larger numbers of patients. Novel strategies with ablative doses of RT may be able to accomplish this goal in patients with inoperable tumors. This review presents the rationale for intensified local therapy with RT using novel techniques that enable the safe delivery of definitive ablative RT doses that commonly are used in other solid tumors. These techniques have the potential to transform the standard management of PDAC.

USE OF VERY AGGRESSIVE SURGICAL RESECTION IN LOCALLY ADVANCED PANCREATIC DUCTAL ADENOCARCINOMA

The role for surgery in PDAC has remained unquestioned as a central necessity in the management of this disease. The consistent belief that margin-negative surgical resection can achieve a cure in this malignancy has led to increasingly aggressive attempts to completely remove the tumor.[9] The Whipple procedure, which is commonly done for pancreatic head tumors, is one of the most complex surgical procedures that can be performed. This is significantly heightened when complex vascular reconstructions are included. Operative times can extend to more than 10 hours, and rates of perioperative morbidity and mortality can increase significantly with complex vascular reconstructions. Series describing these types of surgeries are nearly uniformly retrospective and relatively small in nature. In an example of 1 such series, Zhang and colleagues[10] describe a total of 21 cases of complex vascular resection performed over 6 years. In this series, 18 of the 21 patients recovered without complications; however, 3 patients died from intra-abdominal hemorrhage. Median postoperative survival was 11.6 months. There are several additional retrospective series that have described outcomes of highly complex vascular resections. Notable is that long-term OS is poor, and postoperative mortality high. In some series, these mortality rates can range from 5% to 17%.[11–14] Given the considerable rate of postoperative mortality noted in several of these retrospective series, the oncologic rationale for this strategy is unclear. In patients with such a high propensity for the development of distant metastatic disease, are such aggressive surgical resection attempts truly warranted and helpful?

The high probability for complications coexists with a high probability of distant metastatic disease recurrence. For this reason, the role of arterial resection, for instance, remains controversial. A meta-analysis concluded that such procedures should be considered only at high-volume experienced centers in the context of a clinical trial.[15] When conducted at high-volume centers, outcomes can be excellent.[16] Although in some series, perioperative complications and distant metastatic disease recurrence rates are high in these cases, these complex operations are performed because surgery currently is the only established modality that can achieve long-term disease control and survival. Until a consistently curative local modality is developed, complex surgical resection with vascular resections and reconstruction likely will remain a reasonable consideration. Most surgical oncologists recognize, however, that anatomic complexity and aggressive tumor biology are a bad combination and carefully select patients with locally advanced tumors for surgery. **Table 1** summarizes select series that have published outcomes with more aggressive advanced surgical techniques.

NOVEL STRATEGIES WITH RADIATION THERAPY, ABLATION, AND ADAPTIVE NORMAL TISSUE AVOIDANCE

Image-guided radiation techniques are evolving and converging to enable the ability to address the most significant limitation of the delivery of curative RT doses in the upper abdomen: respiratory, peristaltic, and random motion of the gastrointestinal (GI) tract during radiation delivery. When these challenges are effectively addressed, ablative doses are possible. Historically, doses of RT given for PDAC have been restricted to palliative and adjuvant doses that are incapable of long-term local disease control. The evolution of stereotactic treatment delivery enabled highly conformal and well-tolerated treatment to be given, sometimes with solutions for respiratory motion, but 50% dose reductions from an ablative threshold were necessary due to an inability to account for day-to-day GI motion. Commonly prescribed regimens (25–35 Gy given over 5 fractions) have not produced improved survival duration over conventional regimen (30 Gy given over 10 fractions or 50.4–54 Gy given over 28–30 fractions)[5,17,18] and are biologically similar. All these RT regimens are palliative with no demonstrated survival improvement over chemotherapy alone for inoperable tumors.[5,17] Nearly all other tumors treated curatively with chemotherapy and RT, or definitive RT, are on the order of twice the dose of palliative or adjuvant RT. Higher doses of RT without the use of specialized tools to protect the GI tract have generated poor results due to unacceptable doses to critical local normal structures with resultant bleeding and or perforation.[19] These results have led the field in a direction of maximizing protection of the GI tract, while at the same time increasing the radiation dose to an ablative threshold with a widening of the therapeutic index on both ends.

Novel Methods of Radiation Therapy Delivery

In the past several years, highly novel methods of RT delivery have emerged that will improve the therapeutic index of RT. These novel methods have centered largely around image guidance and improved ability to adapt RT doses to account for the variable location of GI organs from day to day.[20] This approach with RT is often referred to as "adaptive RT," secondary to the ability to change (or adapt) the distribution of RT dose to avoid organs, such as the stomach and jejunum that move in real time. **Fig. 1** illustrates a patient treated with adaptive RT for PDAC with real-time magnetic resonance (MR) guidance. It can be seen that the precise location of organs, such as the stomach, small bowel, and colon, can be visualized daily. These methods have enabled ablative doses of RT to be given safely. By protecting the GI tract from late toxicity (bleeding), MR adaptive delivery secondarily reduces acute toxicities that are related to the doses delivered to the GI tract. **Fig. 2** visually

Table 1
Series on complex vascular reconstructions

Series	N	Vascular Resection/Outcomes Quoted
Sato et al,[13] 2017	10	• Left gastric artery–reconstructing distal pancreatectomy with celiac axis resection. Middle colic artery was used for reconstruction. • Three different reconstruction strategies: left branch reconstruction, right branch reconstruction, and reverse reconstruction • R0 resection was 70%, no ischemic; 9/10 patients underwent adjuvant chemotherapy
Li et al,[12] 2004	79	• Center reporting outcomes of patients who underwent pancreatectomy with vascular reconstruction • A few vascular reconstructions included the superior mesenteric artery or hepatic artery. • Mortality rate was 5%. • Resected endothelia and vascular margins were free of tumor. • Vascular resection (for carefully selected patients) was concluded to be safe and reliable.
Stitzenberg et al,[14] 2008	12	• Median survival after diagnosis was 20 mo. • Median survival after resection was 17 mo (range 1–36 mo). • The 60-d mortality was 17%. • Aggressive surgical approach did not result in any long-term survivors.
Chatzizacharias et al,[16] 2018	108	• Forty-seven (49%) of 96 patients were taken to surgery. • Forty (42%) patients underwent successful resection (28 [62%] of 45 type A and 12 [24%] of 51 type B). • R0 resection was achieved in 32 (80%). • Metastatic disease was found intraoperatively (6 at laparoscopy and 1 at laparotomy) in 7 (15%) of 47 patients. • There were no mortalities; 6 (15%) patients experienced major postoperative complications.
Amano et al,[11] 2009	23	• Median operating time was 686 min (416–1190 min). • Operative mortality was 4.3%. • The 1-y survival was 51.2%. • The 3-y survival was 23.1%. • Median survival time was poor (10 mo). • Conclusions indicate that clarification is required as to surgical indications and significance of such operations.

(continued on next page)

Table 1 *(continued)*		
Series	N	Vascular Resection/Outcomes Quoted
Mollberg et al,[15] 2011	366	• Meta-analyses • Arterial resections were associated with a significantly increased risk for perioperative mortality (odds ratio 5.04). • Arterial resections were associated with poor short-term and long-term outcomes. • Arterial resection should be done in the context of a clinical trial.

highlights modern era MR-guided imaging compared with low-resolution cone beam CT–based imaging.

In recent years, small, mostly retrospective series have begun to emerge demonstrating promising local tumor control and OS using image-guided ablative RT approaches.[21–23] Review articles dedicated to this topic recently have been published.[24] In summary, this technology is in its infancy, because there are only a few early series that show glimpses of promise, but the data appear to consistently show improved 2-year survival for the first time. This area likely will continue to develop until the ideal goal of a continuously changing radiation dose that adapts to movement of the GI organs in real time is realized. When this ideal is approached, comparative trials will be feasible. **Table 2** presents an overview of recent series implementing these RT techniques.

OTHER NOVEL NONSURGICAL LOCAL APPROACHES

In addition to ablative and adaptive image-guided RT, there are novel technologies emerging that may offer potential options for patients with PDAC. Local therapies to have been tested (outside of surgery and RT) include high-frequency ultrasound,[29] radiofrequency ablation,[30] cryotherapy,[31] and irreversible electroporation (IRE).[32] A

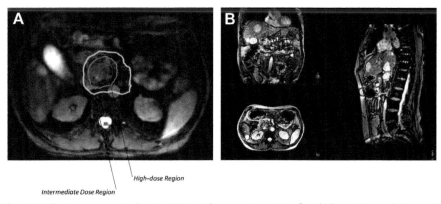

Fig. 1. Daily image acquired using MR guidance, accounting for daily position of the small bowel. (*A*) Daily adapted RT dose. (*B*) Real-time imaging during beam on (*axial, coronal, and sagital view*).

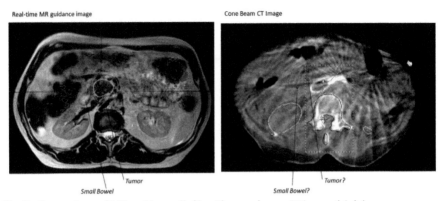

Real-time MR guidance image   Cone Beam CT Image

Tumor
Small Bowel

Tumor?
Small Bowel?

Fig. 2. Comparison of MR guidance (*left*) with cone beam CT image (*right*).

comprehensive review of each of these modalities is beyond the scope of this discussion. One technique that has garnered particular interest is IRE. This also is the subject of a randomized trial comparing it directly to RT (CROSSFIRE; NCT02791503). IRE is an ablative technique that does not involve heat. Instead, IRE involves targeted millisecond, high-voltage electrical pulses that induce cell membrane permeability. This causes defects on the nanoscale in the lipid bilayer of the cell membrane. This results in apoptosis and eventually cell death.[32] Important to recognize is that some series that have used IRE reflect a durable local control and survival in highly selected patients. As with any novel technology, however, there is a significant learning curve associated with this technology. Some early series have seen exceeding high complication rates. As an example, Måansson and colleagues[33] presented their experience with 24 patients with locally advanced PDAC who were treated using percutaneous ultrasound-guided IRE under general anesthesia. Median OS after IRE was 13.3 months compared with 9.9 months in a contemporary registry group. Of the 24 patients, 6 had severe complications following IRE, leading to the conclusion that there were no obvious gains in IRE with first-line treatment of locally advanced PDAC.[33] Despite the potential for a high rate of complications reported in some series, other series have illustrated a relatively high rate of treatment success and, despite complications, have achieved impressive median OSs. An example of such a positive outcome was reported by Narayanan and colleagues in a series of 50 patients with locally advanced PDAC who were treated with percutaneous CT-guided IRE. Despite a relatively high rate of complications, with severe adverse events occurring in 20% of patients, including abdominal pain, pancreatitis, sepsis, and gastric leak, the median OS was 27 months. Patients with tumors less than 3 cm had an even longer median OS of 33 months. This clearly reflects that there are tails to these curves in several different local therapies and that, with effective local control, OS can be extended in this malignancy. The key is to develop understanding of how to optimally achieve durable long-term control while not substantially having an impact on toxicity. Additionally, long-term OS remains poor with a high rate of distant metastatic disease.

RATIONALE TO INCLUDING RADIATION THERAPY IN BORDERLINE RESECTABLE TUMORS

When considering aggressive local interventions in patients with PDAC, there are several key aspects of the disease that should form the foundation for treatment recommendations. First is that distant metastatic disease kills a majority of these

Table 2
Summary of currently published modern era image guided ablative dosing series

Series	N	Methods/Outcomes
Krishnan et al,[25] 2016	200	• Single institution, retrospective • Induction chemotherapy followed by chemotherapy-RT • Range of dose fractionation schedules (63/28, 70/28, 67.5/15, 60/10, and 50/5) • Patients who received BED >70 Gy had a superior OS (17.8 mo vs 15.0 mo; $P = .03$). • Minimal toxicity, grade 1 nausea, vomiting, diarrhea, or fatigue was seen in 37 patients (80%); grade 2 abdominal pain, diarrhea, anorexia, nausea, or fatigue in 13 patients (28%); and grade 3 diarrhea in 1 patient (2%); 4 patients required transfusion. • Radiation dose escalation, done in a highly experienced center, improves OS.
Rudra et al,[23] 2019	44	• Multi-institutional, 5 centers, retrospective • Variety of systemic therapies, including FOLFIRINOX, Gem alone, and FOLFOX, typically given before adaptive MR-guided RT • Grade 3 or higher GI toxicity occurred in 7% of patients. • Patients treated with high-dose RT (BED >70) had improved OS. • A 2-y OS of 49% compared with 30% • Adaptive MR guidance can result in improved OS, with low toxicity, across multiple centers.
Hassanzadeh et al, 2020[26]	44	• Single-institution, retrospective • Late toxicity consisted of 2 (4.6%) grade 3 (GI ulcers) and 3 (6.8%) grade 2 toxicities. • Median OS was 15.7 mo. • The 1-y and 2-y OS rates were 68.2% and 37.9%, respectively.
Chuong et al,[27] 2020	35	• Single-institution, retrospective • Mid-inspiration breath hold, MR guidance • 50 Gy in 5 fractions • The 1-year LC, distant metastasis–free survival, progression-free survival, cause-specific survival, and OS were 87.8%, 63.1%, 52.4%, 77.6%, and 58.9%, respectively.

(continued on next page)

Table 2 (continued)		
Series	**N**	**Methods/Outcomes**
		• Minimal severe treatment toxicity was observed and encouraging local control.
Reyngold et al,[28] 2019	136—primary 33—recurrent	• Single institution, prospective registry • Range of fractionation schedules (75/25, 67.5/15, and 50/5) • Median follow-up of 12 mo • In the primary cohort, median FFLP and OS were not met. • Two-year FFLP and 2-y OS were 76% and 71%, respectively. • Toxicity included grade 3 GI hemorrhage (5%), grade 2 vertebral body fractures (3%), grade 3 bile duct stenosis (2%), and finally grade 2 duodenal ulcer (1%).

Abbreviations: BED, biologically equivalent dose; FFLP, freedom from local progression; LC, local control.

patients. Although approximately a third may die of progressive local/regional issues, a majority will die of poorly controlled distant metastatic disease.[34] Therefore, minimizing time off of systemic therapy needs to be a priority. A modality that can be done quickly (over the course of a few weeks) with a low risk of complications that will prohibit additional systemic therapy is a high priority. Also, a local therapy that provides synergy with surgery also is helpful. Fortunately, RT has been shown in multiple series to accomplish both of these critical tasks. As an example, the Massachusetts General Hospital group demonstrated that total neoadjuvant therapy for patients with locally advanced PDAC can result in a high rate of downstaging and R0 resections in approximately 60% of such patients.[35] Moreover, in multiple analyses, the use of RT consistently has been shown to result in fewer local recurrence events, improved tumor downstaging, improved rates of margin negativity, and less node positivity compared with chemotherapy alone.[36,37] Neoadjuvant RT often can be done effectively over the course of a few weeks and easily interdigitated between cycles of chemotherapy. Modern RT typically is well tolerated and only rarely causes issues with biliary strictures or other toxicities that prohibit chemotherapy administration. In addition, there have been shown to be marginal misses associated with neoadjuvant stereotactic body RT (SBRT) techniques that have attempted to treat just the tumor. These approaches have not covered the volume at risk in the same way that traditional RT techniques have.[38] If advanced technology is used in a neoadjuvant setting, multiple target volumes intended to address not only gross tumor but also areas of microscopic perineural and lymphatic spread are critical. Use of larger RT volumes, treated to intermediate doses, likely will represent an important standard moving forward.

DISCUSSION REGARDING ABLATIVE DOSING OF RADIATION THERAPY VERSUS VERY AGGRESSIVE SURGERY

When considering options for patients with locally advanced PDAC and weighing a very aggressive surgical approach compared with a novel/aggressive RT approach, the data are relatively limited to make this comparison. Certain approaches with RT, including nonadaptive, fiducial-based, CT-guided SBRT, have been shown ineffective in a broad oncology community, such as the US National Clinical Trials Network.[6,39]

Reyngold and colleagues[40] presented 1 such series that raised this consideration in large number of patients treated with ablative RT with favorable OS at 2 years and 3 years. A subsequent comparative analysis from the same institution compared these patients to a group of patients with vascular involvement whose tumors were resected. Despite a selection bias that naturally favored the surgical group, the OS durations were statistically similar. Longer follow-up and greater numbers of patients are needed before definitive conclusions can be made regarding the outcomes of patients beyond 2 years. Both approaches require significant experience and attention to technical details.

SUMMARY

In summary, RT is rapidly evolving and will continue to rapidly evolve in the coming years. The historic techniques associated with RT are being replaced with novel methods of delivering RT. These techniques effectively address the primary limitation that prevents the routine use of ablative RT doses in the upper abdomen, organ motion. Increasingly sophisticated technologies are enabling more and more conformal doses of RT that can be adapted in real time. Such developments will continue to see improvement in outcomes in the coming decade that likely will be dramatic. Artificial intelligence and neural network–based learning will improve the ability to perform daily real-time adaption.[41] Increasingly sophisticated imaging will help identify perineural spread as well as the precise location of the tumor. All these technologies must be kept in mind and considered for their potential to improve outcomes in this devastating malignancy. Clinical trials are needed to robustly evaluate these novel advances as they emerge. The future of adaptive RT is very promising and has direct implications for patients with PDAC.

CLINICS CARE POINTS

- Local recurrence is an extremely common event when patients are treated with surgery first or with chemotherapy alone.
- Clinical outcomes when using chemotherapy and surgery alone for pancreatic cancer are poor when patients are enrolled prior to surgical resection.
- RT is changing dramatically and its important role in the management of pancreatic cancer needs to be considered carefully by surgical oncologists.

DISCLOSURE

Medical College of Wisconsin receives research and travel support from Elekta AB, Stockholm, Sweden.

FUNDING

The project described was supported by the National Center for Advancing Translational Sciences, National Institutes of Health, Award Number KL2TR001438. The content is solely the responsibility of the author(s) and does not necessarily represent the official views of the NIH.

REFERENCES

1. Siegel RL, Miller KD, Jemal A. Cancer statistics, 2020. CA Cancer J Clin 2020; 70(1):7–30.
2. Neoptolemos JP, Palmer DH, Ghaneh P, et al. Comparison of adjuvant gemcitabine and capecitabine with gemcitabine monotherapy in patients with resected pancreatic cancer (ESPAC-4): a multicentre, open-label, randomised, phase 3 trial. Lancet 2017;389(10073):1011–24.
3. Sohal DPS, Duong M, Ahmad SA, et al. Efficacy of Perioperative Chemotherapy for Resectable Pancreatic Adenocarcinoma: A Phase 2 Randomized Clinical Trial. JAMA Oncol 2021;7(3):421–7. https://doi.org/10.1001/jamaoncol.2020.7328.
4. Feig C, Gopinathan A, Neesse A, et al. The pancreas cancer microenvironment. Clin Cancer Res 2012;18(16):4266–76.
5. Hammel P, Huguet F, van Laethem JL, et al. Effect of chemoradiotherapy vs chemotherapy on survival in patients with locally advanced pancreatic cancer controlled after 4 months of gemcitabine with or without erlotinib: the LAP07 randomized clinical trial. JAMA 2016;315(17):1844–53.
6. Katz MH, Shi Q, Meyers JP, et al. Alliance A021501: preoperative mFOLFIRINOX or mFOLFIRINOX plus hypofractionated radiation therapy (RT) for borderline resectable (BR) adenocarcinoma of the pancreas. American Society of Clinical Oncology; 2021.
7. Conroy T, Hammel P, Hebbar M, et al. FOLFIRINOX or gemcitabine as adjuvant therapy for pancreatic cancer. N Engl J Med 2018;379(25):2395–406.
8. Uesaka K, Boku N, Fukutomi A, et al. Adjuvant chemotherapy of S-1 versus gemcitabine for resected pancreatic cancer: a phase 3, open-label, randomised, non-inferiority trial (JASPAC 01). Lancet 2016;388(10041):248–57.
9. Younan G, Tsai S, Evans DB, et al. Techniques of vascular resection and reconstruction in pancreatic cancer. Surg Clin North Am 2016;96(6):1351–70.
10. Zhang Q, Wu J, Tian Y, et al. Arterial resection and reconstruction in pancreatectomy: surgical technique and outcomes. BMC Surg 2019;19(1):141.
11. Amano H, Miura F, Toyota N, et al. Is pancreatectomy with arterial reconstruction a safe and useful procedure for locally advanced pancreatic cancer? J Hepatobiliary Pancreat Surg 2009;16(6):850–7.
12. Li B, Chen FZ, Ge XH, et al. Pancreatoduodenectomy with vascular reconstruction in treating carcinoma of the pancreatic head. Hepatobiliary Pancreat Dis Int 2004;3(4):612–5.
13. Sato T, Inoue Y, Takahashi Y, et al. Distal pancreatectomy with celiac axis resection combined with reconstruction of the left gastric artery. J Gastrointest Surg 2017;21(5):910–7.
14. Stitzenberg KB, Watson JC, Roberts A, et al. Survival after pancreatectomy with major arterial resection and reconstruction. Ann Surg Oncol 2008;15(5):1399–406.
15. Mollberg N, Rahbari NN, Koch M, et al. Arterial resection during pancreatectomy for pancreatic cancer: a systematic review and meta-analysis. Ann Surg 2011;254(6):882–93.
16. Chatzizacharias NA, Tsai S, Griffin M, et al. Locally advanced pancreas cancer: staging and goals of therapy. Surgery 2018;163(5):1053–62.
17. Herman JM, Chang DT, Goodman KA, et al. Phase 2 multi-institutional trial evaluating gemcitabine and stereotactic body radiotherapy for patients with locally

advanced unresectable pancreatic adenocarcinoma. Cancer 2015;121(7): 1128–37.

18. Evans DB, Varadhachary GR, Crane CH, et al. Preoperative gemcitabine-based chemoradiation for patients with resectable adenocarcinoma of the pancreatic head. J Clin Oncol 2008;26(21):3496–502.

19. Chauffert B, Mornex F, Bonnetain F, et al. Phase III trial comparing intensive induction chemoradiotherapy (60 Gy, infusional 5-FU and intermittent cisplatin) followed by maintenance gemcitabine with gemcitabine alone for locally advanced unresectable pancreatic cancer. Definitive results of the 2000-01 FFCD/SFRO study. Ann Oncol 2008;19(9):1592–9.

20. Hall WA, Paulson ES, van der Heide UA, et al. The transformation of radiation oncology using real-time magnetic resonance guidance: a review. Eur J Cancer 2019;122:42–52.

21. Crane CH. Hypofractionated ablative radiotherapy for locally advanced pancreatic cancer. J Radiat Res 2016;57(Suppl 1):i53–7.

22. Crane CH, O'Reilly EM. Ablative radiotherapy doses for locally advanced: pancreatic cancer (LAPC). Cancer J 2017;23(6):350–4.

23. Rudra S, Jiang N, Rosenberg SA, et al. Using adaptive magnetic resonance image-guided radiation therapy for treatment of inoperable pancreatic cancer. Cancer Med 2019;8(5):2123–32.

24. Reyngold M, Parikh P, Crane CH. Ablative radiation therapy for locally advanced pancreatic cancer: techniques and results. Radiat Oncol 2019;14(1):95.

25. Krishnan S, Chadha AS, Suh Y, et al. Focal radiation therapy dose escalation improves overall survival in locally advanced pancreatic cancer patients receiving induction chemotherapy and consolidative chemoradiation. Int J Radiat Oncol Biol Phys 2016;94(4):755–65.

26. Hassanzadeh C, Rudra SBA, Hawkins W. Ablative five-fraction stereotactic body radiation therapy for inoperable pancreatic cancer using online mr-guided adaptation. Adv Radiat Oncol 2020;6(1):100506.

27. Chuong MD, Bryant J, Mittauer KE, et al. Ablative 5-fraction stereotactic magnetic resonance-guided radiation therapy with on-table adaptive replanning and elective nodal irradiation for inoperable pancreas cancer. Pract Radiat Oncol 2020; 11(2):134–47.

28. Reyngold M, O'Reilly E, Zinovoy M, et al. Ablative RT results in excellent local control and survival in localized pancreatic cancer. Int J Radiat Oncol Biol Phys 2019;105(1):S206.

29. Ning Z, Xie J, Chen Q, et al. HIFU is safe, effective, and feasible in pancreatic cancer patients: a monocentric retrospective study among 523 patients. Onco Targets Ther 2019;12:1021–9.

30. Larghi A, Rizzatti G, Rimbaş M, et al. EUS-guided radiofrequency ablation as an alternative to surgery for pancreatic neuroendocrine neoplasms: who should we treat? Endosc Ultrasound 2019;8(4):220–6.

31. Luo XM, Niu LZ, Chen JB, et al. Advances in cryoablation for pancreatic cancer. World J Gastroenterol 2016;22(2):790–800.

32. Lafranceschina S, Brunetti O, Delvecchio A, et al. Systematic review of irreversible electroporation role in management of locally advanced pancreatic cancer. Cancers (Basel) 2019;11(11):1718.

33. Månsson C, Brahmstaedt R, Nygren P, et al. Percutaneous irreversible electroporation as first-line treatment of locally advanced pancreatic cancer. Anticancer Res 2019;39(5):2509–12.

34. Iacobuzio-Donahue CA, Fu B, Yachida S, et al. DPC4 gene status of the primary carcinoma correlates with patterns of failure in patients with pancreatic cancer. J Clin Oncol 2009;27(11):1806–13.

35. Murphy JE, Wo JY, Ryan DP, et al. Total neoadjuvant therapy With FOLFIRINOX in combination with losartan followed by chemoradiotherapy for locally advanced pancreatic cancer: a phase 2 clinical trial. JAMA Oncol 2019;5(7):1020–7.

36. Cloyd JM, Chen HC, Wang X, et al. Chemotherapy versus chemoradiation as preoperative therapy for resectable pancreatic ductal adenocarcinoma: a propensity score adjusted analysis. Pancreas 2019;48(2):216–22.

37. Wittmann D, Hall WA, Christians KK, et al. Impact of neoadjuvant chemoradiation on pathologic response in patients with localized pancreatic cancer. Front Oncol 2020;10:460.

38. Kharofa J, Mierzwa M, Olowokure O, et al. Pattern of marginal local failure in a phase II trial of neoadjuvant chemotherapy and stereotactic body radiation therapy for resectable and borderline resectable pancreas cancer. Am J Clin Oncol 2019;42(3):247–52.

39. Katz MH, Ou F-S, Herman JM, et al. Alliance for clinical trials in oncology (ALLIANCE) trial A021501: preoperative extended chemotherapy vs. chemotherapy plus hypofractionated radiation therapy for borderline resectable adenocarcinoma of the head of the pancreas. BMC Cancer 2017;17(1):1–8.

40. Reyngold M, O'Reilly EM, Varghese AM, et al. Association of Ablative Radiation Therapy With Survival Among Patients With Inoperable Pancreatic Cancer. JAMA Oncol 2021;7(5):735–8. https://doi.org/10.1001/jamaoncol.2021.0057.

41. Huynh E, Hosny A, Guthier C, et al. Artificial intelligence in radiation oncology. Nat Rev Clin Oncol 2020;17(12):771–81.

Pancreaticoduodenectomy and Vascular Reconstruction
Indications and Techniques

Kathleen K. Christians, MD*, Douglas B. Evans, MD

KEYWORDS

- Pancreaticoduodenectomy • Vascular resection
- Borderline and locally advanced pancreas cancer • Mesocaval shunt
- Distal splenorenal shunt

KEY POINTS

- Pancreaticoduodenectomy preparation includes careful preoperative review of high-resolution computed tomography or MRI looking for proximal and distal targets, aberrant anatomy, and extent of disease.
- Tumors tracking up the celiac axis need assessment for tumor involvement of the gastro-duodenal artery and left gastric artery.
- Mesocaval shunting allows a safe resection in the setting of cavernous transformation of the portal vein and widely opens the root of the mesentery, allowing complex arterial dissection.

INTRODUCTION

Pancreatic cancer surgery has evolved from being associated with exceedingly high morbidity and unacceptable mortality to being considered increasingly safe in experienced hands. Vascular resection/reconstruction is now standard practice in many high-volume centers and even patients with borderline resectable and locally advanced disease treated with neoadjuvant therapy and resection can now reach median overall survival rates of 35 to 55 months, justifying the risk.[1–4] These operations are among the most complex surgeries undertaken within the abdominal cavity and require careful preparation to ensure success. This article outlines the key anatomy, preparation, and steps of pancreaticoduodenectomy (PD), with special attention to the anatomic nuances and special circumstances that may require unique solutions and technical expertise/innovation.

Department of Surgery, Medical College of Wisconsin, 8701 Watertown Plank Road, Milwaukee, WI 53226, USA
* Corresponding author.
E-mail address: kchristi@mcw.edu

Surg Oncol Clin N Am 30 (2021) 731–746
https://doi.org/10.1016/j.soc.2021.06.011
1055-3207/21/© 2021 Elsevier Inc. All rights reserved.

Diagnosis

Early signs of pancreatic cancer are epigastric or right upper quadrant abdominal pain, acholic stools (often described as loose or chalky in appearance) dark or orange-colored urine and whole-body pruritis. More subtle findings may include new-onset diabetes or the sudden inability to control blood glucose levels after a prior long-standing steady state and no changes in diet or exercise. Patients may also complain of anorexia caused by a change in taste and unexplained weight loss. These symptoms and signs usually prompt imaging before seeing a specialist, and the single-phase computed tomography (CT) most commonly used in emergency departments is inadequate for staging purposes. Instead, a triple-phase, thin-cut, high-resolution pancreas protocol CT with three-dimensional (3D) rendering and curved planar reformats with/without organ subtraction most accurately allows staging of patients with pancreas cancer. MRI can be done in a similar manner using T1 and T2 sequences along with diffusion weighting and magnetic resonance cholangiopancreatography provided the patient can breath hold and tolerate claustrophobia. Pancreatic adenocarcinomas are usually best visualized on CT in the late arterial phase, standing out from the surrounding parenchyma. This late arterial phase along with curved planar and subtracted images also best shows the relationship of the tumor to the arteries involved, whereas the delayed venous phase axial images best define the presence/absence of venous involvement. It is critical that these images be obtained before biliary stenting and/or biopsies of the tumor are performed to avoid inaccurate reads caused by inflammation from an invasive procedure. Our definition of resectable pancreas cancer includes less than or equal to 50% abutment of the portal vein (PV)–superior mesenteric vein (SMV); therefore, vascular resection and reconstruction may span any of the stages of localized, nonmetastatic disease (resectable, borderline resectable, or locally advanced).

Once a mass is suspected, advanced gastroenterology colleagues perform an endoscopic ultrasound to look for a mass, describe its characteristics, define the relationship to the vasculature, and obtain a tissue diagnosis through fine-needle aspiration or core needle biopsy. Importantly, the authors use on-site cytopathologists to give immediate feedback as to the adequacy of the specimen. Endobiliary metal stents are not placed until the diagnosis can be confirmed because their presence can alter the ability to visualize and confirm a tissue diagnosis necessary to begin neoadjuvant therapy. In addition, if the patient is jaundiced and/or the mass location threatens to obstruct the common bile duct and a tissue diagnosis has been obtained, then a metal stent is placed to maintain biliary patency and prevent jaundice during neoadjuvant therapy.

Anatomy

Preprocedural imaging is then studied for the following items:

Veins

1. Proximal and distal venous targets. In the absence of PV thrombosis, the cephalad PV is usually quite durable and of more than acceptable caliber to create an anastomosis. However, the distal/caudal, targets can be more problematic. As a general rule, the caudal SMV should be 1.5 times the diameter of the superior mesenteric artery (SMA) to provide an adequate target with which to sew. The SMV drains the midgut supplied through 2 first-order venous branches. The ileal branch drains the distal small bowel and colon and runs in a caudal-cranial direction. It is larger (10.2 mm) and more robust than the jejunal vein. In contrast, the jejunal (some refer to this as the first jejunal) branch

drains the proximal small bowel and runs either anterior (40%) or posterior (60%) to the SMA in a transverse, tangential manner (**Fig. 1**A, B). It is usually approximately 2.4 mm smaller in diameter relative to the ileal branch.[5] During the course of PD, one or the other of these first-order vein branches may be safely ligated; however, acute ligation of both branches will result in bowel ischemia and death. Our first preference is to sew to the main trunk of the SMV; however, in some cases, the main trunk is absent (5%; see **Fig. 1**C) and/or the tumor has tracked too far caudally such that the entire main trunk of the SMV must be resected. If the confluence of the ileal and jejunal branches can be preserved, the authors sew to both branches as one (**Fig. 2**). This procedure can be challenging given the posterior trajectory of the jejunal vein, which can skew the anastomosis during creation and/or kink the anastomosis if not aligned correctly. If 1 of these 2 first-order branches requires sacrifice, it is our preference to sew to the ileal branch given the larger diameter and cranial-caudal direction.

2. Location of the splenic vein (SV) –PV-SMV confluence. If possible, based on tumor location, the authors try to preserve the portal-splenic (PV-SV) confluence (**Fig. 3**A). Although this may mean that interposition grafting becomes necessary (**Fig. 3**B), given that the PV-SMV mobility will be diminished with the SV in place, we have found that preservation of flow through this large-caliber SV helps ensure patency of the portal venous system and prevents future development of sinistral portal hypertension.

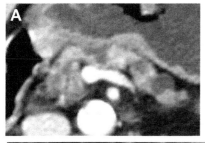
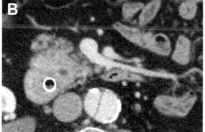
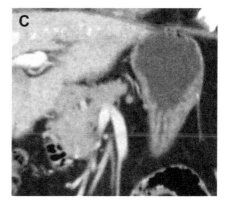

Fig. 1. (*A*) Venous phase axial CT showing an anteriorly located (relative to the SMA) first jejunal vein branch, a less common variant that is associated with further venous abnormalities. (*B*) Venous phase axial CT of a posteriorly located (relative to the SMA) first jejunal vein branch, which is the most common location for this first-order branch. Note the tangential direction and smaller caliber, which make sewing to this in venous resection/reconstruction more difficult than the ileal branch, which runs caudal-cranial and is larger in diameter. (*C*) Venous phase coronal CT showing a venous anomaly where the patient lacks a common SMV trunk but the ileal and jejunal branches emanate from the confluence with the PV–splenic vein. (*Courtesy of* Medical College of Wisconsin.)

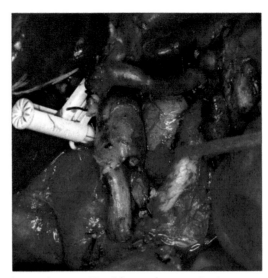

Fig. 2. This patient has undergone PD with vascular resection/reconstruction to the confluence of the ileal and jejunal vein branches. Note the robust caudal-cranial trajectory of the ileal branch and the tangential and posteriorly located (relative to the SMA) jejunal branch. Anastomosis in this location is more difficult because of the trajectory of the vessels but restores venous outflow from the midgut. (*Courtesy of* Medical College of Wisconsin.)

3. Location of inferior mesenteric vein (IMV). Complete evaluation of the preoperative imaging must include location of the IMV. This point is especially important in cases where the PV-SV-SMV confluence is involved and, by definition, in such cases, the SV needs to be ligated for tumor removal. During the process of PD with resection of the PV-SV-SMV confluence, the SV, right

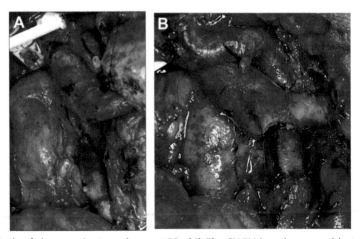

Fig. 3. Both of these patients underwent PD. (*A*) The SV-PV junction was able to be preserved, the first jejunal was ligated because it was engulfed in tumor, and the ileal branch was diverted into the inferior vena cava as a permanent mesocaval shunt. (*B*) More than 2 cm of vein needed to be resected, necessitating interposition grafting with internal jugular vein graft. (*Courtesy of* Medical College of Wisconsin.)

gastroepiploic vein, and often the left gastric veins are ligated acutely, rendering no outflow to the left venous system (stomach and spleen). Over time, this can result in gastroesophageal varices and hemorrhage.[6] In these circumstances, we perform a splenorenal shunt as described by Warren and colleagues[7] (see steps later: special circumstances 1). We do not leave a ligated SV in the absence of decompression from the IMV. If the IMV does not decompress the SV, we perform a splenorenal bypass.

Arteries

Importantly, if an artery is 360° encased, we consider this unresectable (assuming it cannot be resected/reconstructed) because the surgeon would have to cut through tumor to remove it, an oncologically unattractive maneuver. In addition, our group does not recommend resecting/reconstructing the SMA because the risk for bowel ischemia and death can be significant and the complete devascularization of the midgut often results in debilitating diarrhea and nutritional depletion, a quality of life that may make the treatment worse than the disease.

1. Location of the right and common hepatic arteries. The right hepatic artery (RHA) is essential to locate on preoperative imaging. The standard location of the RHA is emanating from the proper hepatic artery (PHA) as an extension from the celiac axis to the common hepatic artery (CHA) to the PHA, and then traveling either posterior or anterior to the common hepatic duct (CHD). In this location, the RHA is usually out of harm's way other than during transection of the bile duct. However, in the setting of a replaced right hepatic artery, the vessel can be replaced from the SMA (**Fig. 4**A), from the celiac axis (**Fig. 4**B), or the entire CHA/PHA/RHA can emanate from the SMA, otherwise known as type IX arterial anatomy (**Fig. 4**C). Inadvertent ligation of a replaced right hepatic artery during PD not only diminishes arterial flow to the right lobe of the liver with risk for abscess but also compromises flow to the bile duct and, therefore, the hepaticojejunostomy used for reconstruction during PD. If type IX arterial anatomy is not recognized and the CHA inadvertently injured, then the liver loses all arterial flow, which can lead to liver necrosis, abscess formation, and future multifocal biliary strictures.

2. Location of the gastroduodenal artery (GDA) relative to the tumor. The GDA emanates from the CHA at the junction with the PHA. The main trunk then courses anterior to the pancreas on the lateral (rightward) aspect of the pancreatic neck. Involvement of the GDA is common in tumors of the pancreatic head and neck. Tumors also frequently track up the GDA to the level of the CHA and PHA, making ligation of the GDA potentially treacherous, especially if radiation is part of the neoadjuvant treatment plan. Following radiation, vessels can be fragile, and indelicate handling of the CHA can result in an inadvertent arterial dissection and resultant ischemia. When the GDA is involved to the level of the CHA/PHA, proximal control is obtained on the CHA such that the origin of the GDA can be carefully sutured closed without the presence of an arterial pressure head.

3. Assess for presence of perineural invasion. Perineural invasion has been found in 80% to 100% of surgical specimens obtained with a surgery-first approach (no neoadjuvant therapy) to pancreatic cancer.[8,9] Perineural invasion is readily visible on appropriately obtained CT imaging sequences, seen as soft tissue tracking along and abutting or encasing the vasculature (**Fig. 5**A). Although the authors preoperatively routinely treat these areas of perineural invasion with radiation, these areas are surgically completely removed en bloc with the specimen. This removal is either done by resecting the involved vessel if necessary or, more commonly, by developing the plain between the adventitia of the artery and the perineurium of the

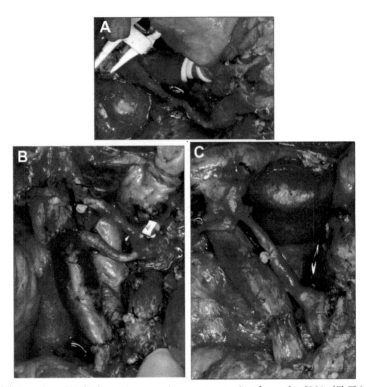

Fig. 4. (A) A replaced right hepatic artery is seen emanating from the SMA. (B) This patient required PV interposition grafting and skeletonization of the celiac axis and SMA for a pancreatic neck tumor. Note a replaced right hepatic artery exiting the right base of the celiac axis. (C) A patient with type IV arterial anatomy in which the CHA arises from the SMA. This patient also required vein resection/reconstruction with primary anastomosis. (*Courtesy of* Medical College of Wisconsin.)

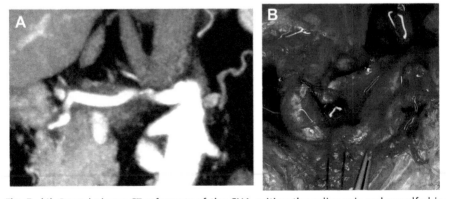

Fig. 5. (A) Curved planar CT reformats of the CHA exiting the celiac axis and engulfed in perineural tumor invasion. (B) The perineural tissue dissected from the CHA that was involved by tumor. This tissue was dissected from the adventitia of the vessel and removed en bloc with the specimen. If this plane cannot be developed, the CHA would be replaced with reversed saphenous vein graft. (*Courtesy of* Medical College of Wisconsin.)

vessel, thereby separating the two and removing this perineurium en bloc with the specimen (**Fig. 5**B). Failure to do so leaves the patient with an R1 (or possibly R2) resection and, by definition, persistence of local disease, which provides no surgical benefit to the patient.

4. Tumors tracking up the celiac axis. Although more commonly seen in the setting of pancreatic body/tail tumors, which is the subject of another article in this issue, some pancreatic neck tumors not only involve the PV-SMV but also track posterior and cephalad along the CHA to the celiac axis. In this clinical scenario, it is imperative to locate both the GDA, which supplies the right gastroepiploic (greater curvature of the stomach), and the left gastric artery (LGA) as it relates to the tumor. If the GDA is involved, then the LGA must be preserved and vice versa; otherwise, the patient is at risk for needing a total gastrectomy in addition to total pancreatectomy, which is something our group does not advocate for adenocarcinoma of the pancreas. The combination of total gastrectomy and total pancreatectomy in the same patient may be nutritionally incompatible with life. Instead, whenever possible, involvement of branches of the celiac axis is handled in one of 2 ways. First, we assess for preservation of the LGA. The distal LGA can be readily located by elevating the stomach cephalad, localizing the pulse and microdissecting the vessel proximally toward its origin from the celiac axis. If the LGA exits the celiac proximal to the junction with the CHA and splenic artery, it often can, and should, be preserved.[10] If it cannot be preserved based on tumor infiltration and the CHA also has to be sacrificed, then the SMA assumes the burden of perfusing the liver retrograde through reverse flow feeding the PHA as well as the right gastroepiploic artery to the stomach. Although this can be done, we do not recommend relying on reversed flow through the SMA alone. We prefer to return flow (supercharge) the CHA either through a primary anastomosis (celiac trunk to redundant residual CHA; **Fig. 6**A) or through a reversed saphenous vein graft from celiac trunk to distal CHA if a long segment of the CHA needs to be removed or lacks redundancy to

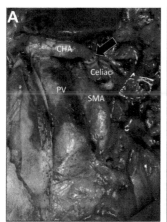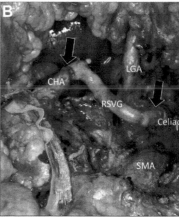

Fig. 6. (*A*) A resected locally advanced tumor shows a skeletonized celiac axis with a ligated LGA and a primary end-to-end anastomosis of the celiac trunk to a redundant CHA. (*B*) This patient also had a locally advanced tumor involving the celiac axis but the LGA was able to be dissected free, thus maintaining excellent arterial flow to the stomach. The proximal CHA had to be resected because of tumor involvement and was reconstructed with reversed saphenous vein graft. RSVG, reversed saphenous vein graft. (*Courtesy of* Medical College of Wisconsin.)

reach the celiac trunk without tension (**Fig. 6**B). This technique restores forward flow both to the liver (CHA) as well as the stomach (GDA–right gastroepiploic), preventing both hepatic ischemia and gastric atony when both the LGA and a segment of the CHA require resection.

Preoperative (Neoadjuvant) Therapy and Surgery

Patients with pancreatic head/neck tumors undergoing PD or extended PD are treated with neoadjuvant chemotherapy (most commonly FOLFIRNOX or gemcitabine-nabpaclitaxel), most often as part of a clinical trial. If restaging reveals a lack of improvement in symptoms, growth in the tumor and/or failed decline in carbohydrate antigen 19-9 (CA 19-9), then the systemic therapy is often changed. In the event of local disease progression, the authors transition to local-regional chemoradiation. Restaging is completed at 2-month intervals (CT scan, laboratories, physical examination, performance status assessment). Usually, after a minimum of 4 months of chemotherapy, patients are transitioned to chemoradiation; a total neoadjuvant approach is currently favored. Our standard is 5.5 weeks of intensity-modulated radiation therapy (IMRT) sensitized by capecitabine or gemcitabine. If the patient is part of our in-house clinical trial comparing IMRT with stereotactic body radiation therapy (SBRT) in the neoadjuvant setting, the patient may potentially be randomized to SBRT. The patient receives supportive care throughout neoadjuvant therapy, including fluids, growth factor support, regular visits with our pancreatic dietitians, and nutritional supplementation. Following the conclusion of neoadjuvant therapy, the patient is started on a course of prehabilitation through physical therapy and receives nutritional shakes to boost nutrition and supplement the immune system. They are seen by our preoperative clinic to maximize medical management and also complete any other necessary screening examinations (colonoscopy, mammograms, prostate examination, and so forth) in the intervening time before surgery. We strongly encourage all of our patients to also see our dedicated Pancreatic Cancer Program psychologist for several preoperative visits during neoadjuvant therapy, similar to the experience in college and professional athletics with psychological support for stress management and optimization of the mind-body relationship. Our preference is to then operate between 4 and 6 weeks following the completion of chemoradiation.

The patient receives a light bowel prep the day before surgery; showers the night before and on the morning of surgery, including use of Hibiclens wipes; and remains nothing by mouth after midnight with the exception of a nutritional shake. In the operating room, invasive monitoring includes accessing the existing power port and placing 2 large-bore intravenous (IV) lines and an arterial line. In the setting of anticipated vascular resection/reconstruction, the left neck is prepped and draped, as is the territory of 1 saphenous vein deemed to be of best caliber by preoperative vascular duplex studies. IV antibiotics are administered to cover bowel organisms (usually ceftriaxone and metronidazole, assuming no allergies exist). We prefer to leave both arms out at a 90° angle to the patient's torso and place 1 leg in a frog-leg position with appropriate padding under all extremities. Assuming the left internal jugular vein will be used for interposition graft, the left neck is prepped and the patients face directed slightly toward the right with a small roll placed transversely under the shoulders to better expose territory of the internal jugular vein. The patient is placed on a bed warmer, has a warming blanket over the unused portion of the legs, and has a temperature probe foley catheter placed. Our anesthesiology team includes a dedicated group of certified registered nurse anesthetists who have acquired a significant experience in the perioperative management of patients undergoing complex pancreatic cancer surgery.

Procedural Approach

PD for cancer starts with a diagnostic laparoscopy unless the operative intent is a double bypass (biliary and gastric bypass) for the findings of locally unresectable or metastatic disease. Following a diagnostic laparoscopy devoid of metastases, an upper midline incision is made. As discussed in prior publications, the authors perform PD in a clockwise 6-step manner that includes the following[11,12]:

(1) Elevate the omentum off the transverse colon, widely open up the lesser sac, take down the hepatic flexure of the colon, and expose the infrapancreatic SMV.
(2) Perform an extended Kocher maneuver to the level of the aorta, removing all tissue anterior to the inferior vena cava (IVC) and medial to the right gonadal vein.
(3) Dissect the porta hepatis, including removal of the CHA node, dissection/mobilization of the CHA, PHA, and RHA, and ligation of right gastric artery and the GDA. Once the vascular anatomy is verified, a cholecystectomy is completed and the CHD is transected just cephalad to the cystic duct entrance or mid–common duct if the cystic duct has a high insertion. The hepatic duct is usually transected before ligation of the GDA to further clarify arterial anatomy, especially when the dissection is difficult because of fibrosis, adhesions, or scar.
(4) A modest antrectomy is then performed normally using 2 loads of the gastrointestinal anastomosis stapler. The blood supply to the lesser and greater curvature is ligated along with splitting the omentum at the level of the transection margin with the Ligasure device.
(5) The ligament of Treitz is mobilized, taking care to preserve the IMV, and the jejunum is transected with a stapler. The mesentery to the proximal jejunum/distal duodenum is taken down with a Ligasure device and the bowel is rotated underneath the root of the mesentery into the right upper quadrant. The retroperitoneal leaflet is then taken down with electrocautery to provide bimanual palpation as well as complete mobilization of the head of the pancreas.
(6) Sutures are then placed in the pancreas proximal and distal to the anticipated transection margin (usually pancreatic neck directly overlying the SMV) and the pancreas is transected with electrocautery. The specimen is then dissected from the PV/SMV cephalad to the first jejunal vein branch as well as the SMA, taking care to remove all soft tissue and nerve respectively, along the right anterolateral aspect of these vessels en bloc with the specimen. Portal, retroportal, and retroperitoneal lymphadenectomy is usually then completed after the specimen is removed. En face margins are taken from the biliary and pancreatic margin for frozen section.

Reconstruction

A retrocolic jejunal limb is brought through the bare area of the transverse colon mesentery to the right of the middle colic vessels and sutured end of pancreas to side of jejunum in 2 layers (occasionally 1), usually with interrupted 4-0 or 5-0 polydioxanone (PDS) suture. The inner layer is pancreatic duct to full- thickness enterotomy and the outer layer is interrupted horizontal mattress. Ten centimeters caudal, an end-to-side hepaticojejunostomy is created with a single layer of interrupted PDS suture. Then, 50 to 60 cm distal to the biliary reconstruction, in an antecolic manner, an end-to-side gastrojejunostomy is created. The more cephalad staple line can be oversewn with Lembert sutures and the caudal aspect used for the anastomosis. This procedure can be done either in 1 or 2 layers, and our preference is to sew this anastomosis. The opening in the mesentery where the jejunal limb was brought up for the anastomoses should then either be closed around the jejunum or widely opened to allow free movement of bowel and prevent internal herniation. The bowel is then carefully run and the remaining omentum arranged to avoid torque on the gastrojejunostomy. In addition, the falciform ligament is then draped over the GDA stump, underneath the hepaticojejunostomy and overlying the SMA to prophylactically cover and protect these areas in the event of a pancreatic leak.

Standard Vein Resection/Reconstruction

Whenever possible, the SMA is dissected out in an SMA-first approach, usually by incising along the left side of the SMV (**Fig. 7**). Localizing the SMA first prevents it from being inadvertently injured and also allows for inflow occlusion during SMV-PV clamping. The SMA is encircled with a Rumel tourniquet. The PV above and the SMV below are dissected out with enough distance to both place vascular clamps and to have room to sew. If the confluence is involved by tumor, the SV is ligated. If the confluence is not involved, the SV-PV junction is preserved to improve flow and therefore patency of the PV. The patient is then systemically heparinized, and a mark is placed longitudinally along the 12 o'clock position on both the SMV and PV to maintain orientation while sewing the anastomoses. Any retraction on the

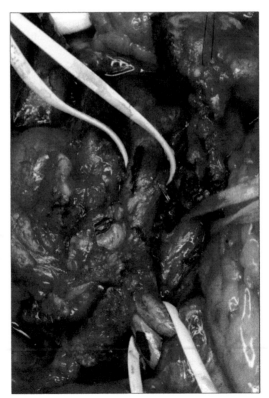

Fig. 7. A distal SMV tumor still attached to the vein. The SMA is dissected out first to prevent injury during vascular resection/reconstruction, otherwise known as an SMA-first approach. (*Courtesy of* Medical College of Wisconsin.)

mesentery is released/lessened. The Rumel tourniquet is then cinched down and the PV and SMV are clamped with straight vascular clamps. The specimen is removed. The SMV is sutured end to end to the left internal jugular vein graft (IJVG) with interrupted 6-0 Prolene and subsequently end to end to the PV with the same technique. Heparinized saline is used before tying the last stitch and the anastomoses are also back bled. The final caudal clamp is released, thereby restoring flow to the liver, and the Rumel tourniquet is removed, restoring arterial flow to the intestines (**Fig. 8**).

Special Circumstance 1: Tumor Involvement of the Confluence, Inferior Mesenteric Vein Draining into SMV

In the setting of tumor involvement at the PV-SV-SMV confluence, ligation of the SV is necessary. If the IMV enters the SMV either at, or caudal to, the confluence (as opposed to the SV), the authors prefer to perform a distal splenorenal shunt (DSRS).[13,14] The authors transect the SV, oversew the portal side with 4-0 or 5-0 Prolene, and meticulously dissect out enough length of the SV from the posterior aspect of the pancreatic body to reach the left renal vein. Dividing the pancreas is usually helpful in mobilizing the distal SV. The left adrenal and renal veins are localized through the mesenteric root, usually caudal to the pancreas and lateral to the SMA. With experience, this can be done with careful dissection and/or with the aid of ultrasonography guidance. The distal SV is then anastomosed to the junction of the left adrenal and left renal vein to complete a DSRS. Specifically, the left adrenal vein is ligated caudally (toward the adrenal gland), and the confluence of the left adrenal and left renal veins are used to create the anastomosis. A side-biting Satinsky clamp is placed on the left renal vein and a baby bulldog on the SV. The posterior wall of the anastomosis is sutured

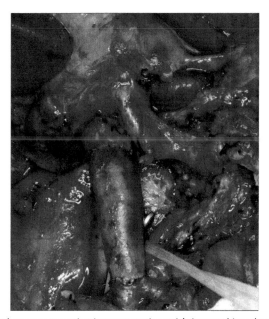

Fig. 8. A completed venous resection/reconstruction with internal jugular vein interposition graft. Note that the internal jugular vein is typically a good size match for this endeavor and uses the patient's own tissue, thereby lessening risk of an infected graft in the event of a leak. (*Courtesy of* Medical College of Wisconsin.)

with a running 6-0 Prolene and the anterior wall with interrupted 6-0 Prolene suture. An interrupted growth stitch is placed at the lateral apex of the anastomosis and tied to the posterior running stitch to prevent narrowing of the anastomosis (**Fig. 9**). Heparinized saline is instilled before tying the last stitch, the anastomosis is back bled, and vascular clamps are then released to restore flow. Creation of this DSRS prevents development of left-sided (sinistral) portal hypertension. An added advantage is that, with the SV no longer tethering the PV-SMV in place, a primary venous anastomosis (SMV to PV) often can be completed rather than the need for interposition grafting.

Special Circumstance 2: Perineural Invasion of the Superior Mesenteric Artery and/or Branches of the Celiac Axis and the Need for Concomitant Venous Resection/Reconstruction or Cavernous Transformation of the Portal Vein

When venous resection/reconstruction is necessary and the tumor tracks up the root of the mesentery to the origin of the SMA and/or to the proximal CHA or the celiac axis (common in pancreatic neck tumors), the authors have found it helpful to use a mesocaval shunt. This technique is also necessary in the setting of cavernous transformation of the PV to prevent exsanguination from varices during pancreatic resection.[14–16]

The lesser sac is opened and the SMV is localized as it emerges from the caudal mesentery. Ideally the vein is localized just cephalad to the takeoff of the jejunal and ileal branches (ie, sew to the confluence of the jejunal and ileal branches or just cephalad on the main trunk of the SMV). An internal jugular vein is usually harvested from the left neck, taking care to maintain the vein's orientation by marking it longitudinally with a marker and noting the cephalad and caudal ends. The IVC was previously dissected out during step 2 of the standard Whipple (extended Kocher maneuver) and the ligament of Treitz is taken down. The devascularized segment of proximal jejunum and distal duodenum is then reflected beneath the SMA/SMV. If possible,

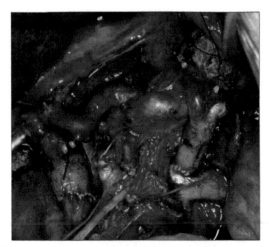

Fig. 9. A DSRS. In this patient, the left coronary vein entered the SV and was also preserved. This DSRS diverts left-sided flow into the renal vein, thereby preventing any potential for sinistral portal hypertension. Note also that moving the SV also then allowed a primary anastomosis of the PV-SMV following venous resection. (*Courtesy of* Medical College of Wisconsin.)

the uncinate process is separated from the SMV and then the SMA. The infrarenal IVC is clamped with a side-biting Satinsky vascular clamp. The IVC is incised with a knife and the end of the left IJVG is sutured to the side of the IVC with running 6-0 Prolene. A small bulldog is placed on the vein graft and the Satinsky is then removed from the IVC. The SMV is clamped with a straight vascular clamp caudally and the cephalad (specimen side) is grasped and the vein is transected. The specimen side is oversewn to prevent back bleeding from the specimen. The caudal SMV is then anastomosed end to end to the proximal end of the IJVG with interrupted 6-0 Prolene suture, thereby creating a mesocaval shunt (IVC-IJVG-SMV; **Fig. 10**A). Heparinized saline is instilled and the graft is perfused before removing the small bulldog clamp just proximal to the IVC anastomosis and releasing forward flow into the IVC (so as to prevent an air embolism). The authors do the IVC anastomosis first to avoid a prolonged clamp time on the SMV and the need for inflow occlusion on the SMA. This maneuver not only decompresses portal collaterals in the setting of cavernous transformation of the PV but also widely opens up the root of the mesentery, allowing a difficult arterial dissection to proceed safely and unimpeded where the tumor would normally obscure the view of this critical anatomy. The remaining specimen dissection is completed (steps 2–6 of the standard Whipple), to include transection of the PV at the superior border of the pancreas, and the specimen is removed. We then prepare for restoration of portal flow (hepatofugal flow). Namely, the patient is systemically heparinized, a Rumel tourniquet on the SMA is cinched down for inflow occlusion to prevent bowel edema, and both SMV and distal IJVG are controlled with small bulldog clamps or straight vascular clamps. The IJVG is then disconnected from the IVC, leaving a small cuff of vein graft to oversew on the IVC. The IJVG is then trimmed to an appropriate length not creating too much laxity or tension and then sutured end to end to the

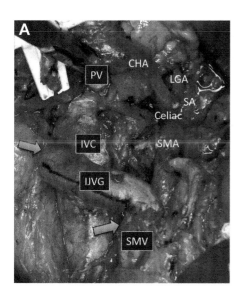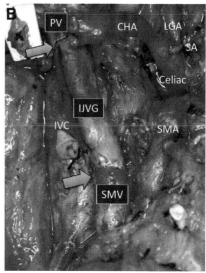

Fig. 10. (*A*) A patient undergoing total pancreatectomy with the initial step using a meso-caval shunt (SMV-IJVG-IVC) to decompress the intestines, making the dissection/resection more hemostatic and widely opening the mesentery, allowing complex dissection of the celiac axis and SMA. (*B*) A ligated mesocaval shunt with the end toward the IVC disconnected and reanastomosed end to end to the cephalad PV, thereby restoring full flow to the liver during total pancreatectomy. (*Courtesy of* Medical College of Wisconsin.)

PV (**Fig. 10**B) Again, heparinized saline and back bleeding of the anastomosis are completed before release of the cephalad and caudal vascular clamps.

Recovery

Following PD vascular resection/reconstruction, the patient is brought to the recovery room usually having been extubated in the operating room. A full set of laboratory tests is obtained, focusing particularly on the arterial blood gas for base deficit, a complete blood count for hemoglobin, hematocrit and platelet count, and International Normalized Ratio (INR). If the platelet count is in the normal range and a vein resection/reconstruction has been completed, the patient receives 300 mg of aspirin, per rectum in recovery, and a daily aspirin thereafter. If the INR is less than 1.5 and the patient has no evidence of ongoing blood loss, 5000 U of subcutaneous heparin is also administered either in recovery or several hours later on the floor following rewarming and stabilization. Most of these patients are managed on a standard surgical oncology ward rather than the intensive care unit by nurses familiar with these postoperative patients; approximately 5% of our patients spend 1 night in the surgical intensive care unit. Although crystalloid resuscitation is standard, albumin boluses are also given freely based on end points of resuscitation (hemodynamics, urine output, base deficit). IV antibiotics are given on induction and redosed for a minimum of 24 to 72 hours depending on the presence/absence of endobiliary stents and guided by intraoperative bile duct cultures taken at the time of bile duct transection. Diabetes management, physical therapy, occupational therapy, and pancreatic dietitians are consulted to help facilitate the patient's postoperative recovery. Patients are allowed clear liquids while a nasogastric tube is in place and then have their diets advanced as the tube is removed and bowel function returns. Drains placed (usually in right gutter to drain ascites and lymph) are removed when outputs diminish, usually around day 3 or 4. Daily calorie counts are calculated until caloric intake is sufficient to allow discharge. Patients with vein resection/reconstruction were previously discharged on aspirin and Lovenox but more recently are released with an oral anticoagulant such as Eliquis (50% dose; 2.5 mg twice a day) and aspirin for patient convenience/compliance and reduced cost.

Outcomes

As our group has previously published, the potential for a patient to complete all intended neoadjuvant therapy (usually to include chemotherapy and radiation) and undergo complete resection varies by disease stage. Those with resectable disease have greater than 90% chance of successfully completing all intended therapy with a median overall survival (OS) of 45 months.[17] Those with borderline resectable disease have a nearly 75% chance of successfully completing all treatment with a resultant median OS of 31 to 38 months, and the highly selected patients with locally advanced type A disease are successfully resected 62% of the time and have a median OS of 56 months, whereas locally advanced type B patients are resected 24% of the time with a median OS of 37.5 months (median OS of both locally advanced groups combined of 39 months).[3,4,18]

SUMMARY

PD in the setting of venous and/or arterial involvement can be done safely following neoadjuvant therapy in experienced hands with careful preoperative planning and attention to key principles of anatomy and operative technique. Standardized protocols and multidisciplinary management both preoperatively and postoperatively optimize patient care and outcomes. Following these standards, patients can expect outcomes 3 times those of historical controls.

DISCLOSURE

None.

REFERENCES

1. Gemenetzis G, Groot VP, Blair AB, et al. Survival in Locally Advanced Pancreatic Cancer After Neoadjuvant Therapy and Surgical Resection. Ann Surg 2019; 270(2):340–7.
2. Michelakos T, Pergolini I, Fernandez-del Castillo, et al. Predictors of Resectability and Survival in Patients With Borderline and Locally Advanced Pancreatic Cancer who Underwent Neoadjuvant Treatment With FOLFIRINOX. Ann Surg 2019; 269(4):733–40.
3. Chatzizacharias N, Tsai S, Griffin M, et al. Locally Advanced Pancreas Cancer – Staging and Goals of Therapy. Surgery 2018 May;163(5):1053–62.
4. Barnes CA, Chavez MI, Tsai S, et al. Survival of patients with borderline resectable pancreatic cancer who received neoadjuvant therapy and surgery. Surgery 2019;166(3):277–85.
5. Papavasiliou P, Arrangoiz R, Zhu F, et al. The anatomic Course of the First Jejunal Branch of the Superior Mesenteric Vein in Relation to the Superior Mesenteric Artery. Int J Surg Oncol. 2012;2012:538769.
6. Pilgrim CHC, Tsai S, Tolat P, et al. Optimal Management of the splenic vein at the time of venous resection for pancreatic cancer: Importance of the inferior mesenteric vein. J Gastrointest Surg 2014;18(5):917–21.
7. Warren WD, Zeppa R, Fomon JJ. Selective trans-splenic decompression of gastroesophageal varices by distal splenorenal shunt. Ann Surg 1967;166(3): 437–55.
8. Chatterjee D, Katz MH, Rashid A, et al. Am J Surg Pathol 2012;36(3):409–17.
9. Schorn S, Demir IE, Haller B, et al. The influence on survival and tumor recurrence in pancreatic ductal adenocarcinoma. Surg Oncol 2017;26(1):105–15.
10. Okada Ki, Kawai M, Tani M, et al. Preservation of the Left Gastric Artery on the Basis of Anatomical Features in Patients Undergoing Distal Pancreatectomy with Celiac Axis En-bloc Resection (DP-CAR). World J Surg 2014;38:2980–5.
11. Christians KK, Tsai S, Tolat P, et al. Critical Steps for Pancreaticoduodenectomy in the Setting of Pancreatic Adenocarcinoma. J Surg Oncol 2013;107(1):33–8.
12. Evans DB, Tolat P, Christians KK. Pancreatectomy (Whipple Operation) and Total Pancreatectomy for Cancer. In: Fischer JL, editor. Mastery of surgery, 127, 7th edition. Philadelphia: Wolters Kluwer/Lippincot Williams & Wilkins; 2018. p. 1552–73.
13. Christians KK, Riggle K, Keim R, et al. Distal Splenorenal and Temporary Mesocaval Shunting at the Time of Pancreatectomy for Cancer: Initial Experience from the Medical College of Wisconsin. Surgery 2013;154(1):123–31.
14. Chavez MI, Tsai S, Clarke CN, et al. Distal splenorenal and mesocaval shunting at the time of pancreatectomy. Surgery 2019;165(2):298–306.
15. Pilgrim C, Tsai S, Evans DB, et al. Mesocaval shunting – a novel technique to facilitate venous resection and reconstruction and enhance exposure of the superior mesenteric and celiac arteries during pancreaticoduodenectomy. J Am Coll Surg 2013;217(3):e17–20.

16. Younan G, Tsai S, Evans DB, et al. Techniques of Vascular Resection and Reconstruction in Pancreatic Cancer. Surg Clin North Am 2016;96(6):1351–70.
17. Christians KK, Heimler JW, George B, et al. *Survival of patients with resectable pancreatic cancer receiving neoadjuvant therapy.* Presented as long oral Pancreas Club 2015. Surgery 2016;159(3):893–900.
18. Tsai S, Christians KK, George B, et al. A Phase II Clinical Trial of Molecular Profiled Neoadjuvant Therapy for Localized Pancreatic Ductal Adenocarcinoma. Ann Surg 2018;268(4):610–9.

Minimally Invasive Techniques for Pancreatic Resection

Ibrahim Nassour, MD, MSCS[a], Alessandro Paniccia, MD[a],
A. James Moser, MD[b], Amer H. Zureikat, MD[c],*

KEYWORDS

- Minimally invasive • Robotic • Pancreaticoduodenectomy • Whipple
- Distal pancreatectomy

KEY POINTS

- Minimally invasive pancreaticoduodenectomy (MIPD) should only be performed in highly specialized centers and following stringent training to assure optimal outcomes.
- There are four randomized trials comparing laparoscopic versus open pancreaticoduodenectomies with mixed results.
- Minimally invasive surgery is the standard of care for all benign and most malignant left pancreatic pathologies.
- There are two randomized trials comparing minimally invasive versus open distal pancreatectomies favoring the minimally invasive approach.

INTRODUCTION

Minimally invasive surgery (MIS) has been widely adopted in multiple surgical disciplines but has remained underutilized in surgical oncology in general—and pancreatic surgery in particular—because of the complexity of the operations and their high morbidity. Over the last decade, the enthusiasm to adopt this technique has been reinforced by the creation of training programs and a more systematic implementation of this approach.[1–11] In 2019, the Miami international evidence-based guidelines on minimally invasive pancreas resection supported the use of minimally invasive distal pancreatectomy (MIDP) but acknowledged that there is insufficient data to recommend minimally invasive pancreaticoduodenectomy (MIPD) over the open

Funding: none.
Conflicts of interest: nothing to declare.
[a] University of Pittsburgh Medical Center, Pittsburgh, PA, USA; [b] Harvard Medical School, Pancreas and Liver Institute, Beth Israel Deaconess Medical Center, Boston, MA 02215, USA; [c] Division of Surgical Oncology, University of Pittsburgh Medical Center, 5150 Center Avenue, Suite 421, Pittsburgh, PA 15232, USA
* Corresponding author.
E-mail address: zureikatah@upmc.edu

approach.[12] In this review, we present the important criteria to consider when selecting a patient for minimally invasive pancreatic surgery, describe the technical aspects of both robotic pancreaticoduodenectomy (RPD) and robotic distal pancreatectomy (RDP), and focus on prospective and large retrospective studies that describe the outcomes following minimally invasive pancreatic surgery. As the authors' expertise is mainly in the robotic approach to pancreatectomy, selection criteria, learning curve, and technical details of RPD and RDP will be emphasized.

PATIENT SELECTION

Careful patient selection is paramount to assure the safety and success of the minimally invasive approach, especially during the early learning curve. Although the indications for minimally invasive approach are similar to the open approach, the following considerations should be taken into account:

1. Preoperative staging with a pancreatic protocol triphasic computed tomography scan is essential for MIS patient selection. Tumors in the head of the pancreas with vascular involvement or those with replaced or aberrant arterial anatomy are best approached open, especially as the surgical team is working through the MIS learning curve. Tumors in body/tail tumor involving branches of the celiac axis should have no disease at the celiac trunk or the gastroduodenal artery (GDA) so that a distal pancreatectomy with en bloc resection of the celiac axis is feasible.
2. Periampullary nonpancreatic tumors represent the ideal case for resection but pose significant challenges in reconstruction due to soft pancreata and small nondilated pancreatic and biliary ducts. Ideal cases for early adopters are small pancreatic ductal adenocarcinomas (PDAC) with both biliary and pancreatic duct obstruction and no vascular involvement. This facilitates a safe resection and reduces the risk of biliary and pancreatic fistulae because of the large size of the ducts and the firm texture of the pancreas. The selection criteria can be expanded to other pathologies once the surgeon becomes more experienced.
3. Patients with extreme body mass index (BMI) can pose challenges for the minimally invasive approach (especially the robotic DaVinci platform approach). Patients with very low BMI will have inadequate space for robotic instruments (ideally one handsbreadth between the robotic ports) and those with high BMI will pose challenges in mobilizing the transverse mesocolon, dividing the ligament Treitz, and exposing the uncinate process.
4. Patients with multiple surgical procedures and extensive adhesions requiring an extended time of lysis should not be offered a minimally invasive approach, which at baseline has a longer operative time than the open approach. In particular, patients with prior upper gastrointestinal reconstruction are best avoided robotically, as lack of haptic feedback may lead to bowel injuries during manipulation.

LEARNING CURVE FOR MINIMALLY INVASIVE PANCREATECTOMY

In addition to stringent selection criteria, surgeons must navigate through the learning curve for minimally invasive pancreatectomy with safe outcomes. In a risk-adjusted CUSUM analysis of the first 200 consecutive RPD, the authors identified several inflexion points in their learning curve experience.[2] Statistical improvements in conversion rates to open surgery and estimated blood loss occurred after 20 cases (35.0% vs 3.3% [$P<.001$] and 600 mL vs 250 mL [$P = .002$], respectively), reduction in the incidence of postoperative pancreatic fistula (POPF) after 40 cases (27.5% vs 14.4%; $P = .04$), and faster operating room times after 80 cases (581 vs 417 minutes

[*P*<.001]). A similar analysis of our first 100 consecutive RDP identified a learning curve of 40 cases needed to optimize operative time and outcomes. The learning curve for laparoscopic pancreatectomy seems to be similar with several reports indicating 40 to 100 cases to reach proficiency.[13–15]

In the authors' view, important considerations to a successful learning curve are:

1. The need for a sufficient experience in open pancreatectomy. As minimally invasive pancreatectomy should follow principles of open surgery, a thorough understanding of relevant anatomy, oncologic principles, and technical tricks and pitfalls of open pancreatectomy allow for safe and efficient implementation of minimally invasive pancreatectomy.
2. Availability of two attendings during the learning curve. This is particularly important for RPD, where two attendings were involved (a bedside and console surgeon operating in tandem) for all initial procedures during the authors' robotic learning curve. This ensures safe outcomes, shared learning, and minimizes "mission creep" for procedures with long learning curves.
3. The learning curve should be preferably completed within a short time frame—in the author's experience, 80 cases within 3 years. We recommend performing 2 to 3 cases per month to allow for rapid assimilation of experience by the surgeons and the operative team as a whole. Similarly, a National Cancer Database (NCDB) analysis revealed that hospitals performing a minimum of 10 laparoscopic pancreaticoduodenectomy (LPD) per year were able to achieve low mortality comparable with open pancreaticoduodenectomy (OPD).[16]
4. Need for dedicated curricula, mentoring, and coursework that can reduce the learning curve for new adopters. At the author's institution, training in robotic pancreatic surgery follows a systematic approach. Both RPD and RDP are broken down into specific steps (7 steps for RPD and 3 for RDP [see below]). Trainees are provided access to a virtual library of robotic pancreatic procedures, enrolled in a virtual reality curriculum (focused on mastery of instruments, controls and endowrist functions), and complete a biotissue curriculum focused on reconstruction drills. Once these are completed, training transitions into the operating room where graduated autonomy is provided based on operative proficiency.

TECHNICAL ASPECTS OF ROBOTIC PANCREATICODUODENECTOMY
Positioning and Port Placement

The patient is positioned supine on a split leg table with the legs abducted to allow for the bedside assistant to stand between the legs. The left arm is placed on an arm board and the right arm is tucked. The patient should be appropriately padded and anchored well to the table with circumferential straps over the chest and legs. The operative table is placed in steep Trendelenburg and the XI robot is docked from the right side of the patient.

Using a 5-mm zero-degree scope and an optical trocar, the abdomen is accessed in the left upper quadrant. The abdomen is insufflated to 15 mm Hg, a diagnostic laparoscopy is performed, and 6 additional ports are placed, as described in **Fig. 1**A. The Mediflex liver retractor is placed through a 5-mm trocar laterally inferior to the left costal margin. The robot is docked (from the right side for XI or over the patient's head for the SI robot), and the operation is started.

The Steps of the Operation

Mobilization of the right colon, Kocherization, and division of the ligament of Treitz
The lesser sac is accessed by taking down the gastrocolic ligament. The adhesions between the pancreas and stomach are taken down and the transverse mesocolon

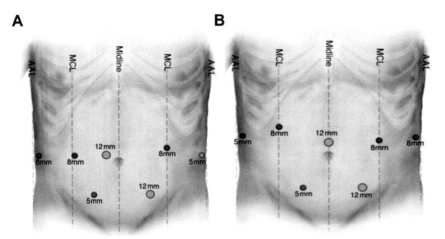

Fig. 1. (*A*) Port configuration for RPD. Robotic ports in the upper abdomen: the camera (*Green*) is placed through a 12 mm port for the SI or 8 mm port for the XI. The three other robotic arms (*Purple*) are 8 mm for the SI and XI (right AAL, right MCL, and left MCL). Laparoscopic ports in the lower abdomen: self-retaining liver retractor (*Blue*) through a 5 mm port in the left AAL, two laparoscopic bedside assistant ports; a 12 mm port (*Green*) in the left lower quadrant and 5 mm port (*Red*) in the right lower quadrant. (*B*) Port configuration for robotic distal pancreatectomy. Robotic ports in the upper abdomen: the camera (*Green*) is placed through a 12 mm port for the SI or 8 mm port for the XI. The three other robotic arms (*Purple*) are 8 mm for the SI and XI (right MCL, left MCL, and left AAL). Laparoscopic ports in the lower abdomen: self-retaining liver retractor (*Blue*) through a 5 mm port in the right AAL, two laparoscopic bedside assistant ports; a 12 mm port (*Green*) in the left lower quadrant and 5 mm port (*Red*) in the right lower quadrant. AAL, anterior axillary line; MCL, midclavicular line.

is dissected inferiorly. After mobilizing the hepatic flexure, the duodenum is Kocherized and the ligament of Treitz is divided. This will allow the duodenum to be completely freed and the proximal jejunum to be delivered in the right supracolic compartment. Using an endo GIA stapler with a 60 mm gold staple load, the proximal jejunum is transected 10 cm from the duodenum. Finally, the jejunal mesentery is resected with the Ligasure from the supracolic compartment up the uncinate.

Division of the stomach and dissection of the porta-hepatis

The gastrohepatic ligament is opened. The right gastric and right gastroepiploic vessels are divided with the Ligasure at the lesser and greater stomach curvatures. Then, the stomach is divided proximal to the pylorus using an endo GIA with a 60 mm purple staple load. Next, the station 8A lymph node is dissected off the common hepatic artery followed by the GDA, portal vein (PV), and common bile duct. The GDA and the common bile duct are transected with an endo GIA stapler using 45 mm gold load (**Fig. 2A**). The GDA is reinforced with a robotic hemlock or laparoscopic 10 mm clip. Finally, the retropancreatic tunnel is started by dissecting the anterior border of the PV off the pancreas using the robotic hook.

Transection of the pancreatic neck

After retracting the duodenum toward the right upper quadrant to create tension on the gastroepiploic vein, the superior mesenteric vein (SMV) is identified, and its anterior surface is dissected. Next, the gastroepiploic vein is divided with the Ligasure and

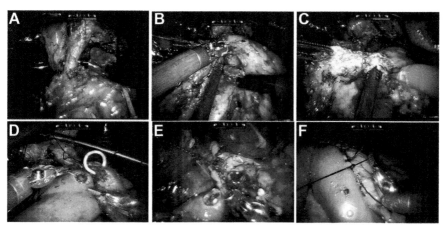

Fig. 2. (*A*) GDA transection. (*B*) Creation of the tunnel between the pancreatic neck and SMV. (*C*) Pancreas transection. (*D*) Pancreaticojejunostomy. (*E*) Hepaticojejunostomy. (*F*) Gastrojejunostomy.

the retropancreatic tunnel is created (**Fig. 2**B). Finally, the parenchyma of the pancreatic neck is divided with hot monopolar shears and the duct is sharply divided (**Fig. 2**C).

Dissection of the uncinate
The uncinate is exposed by retracting the specimen laterally and the fibers between the SMV/PV and the uncinate are divided with a hook cautery. The vein of Belcher is divided superiorly with Ligasure, and the inferior pancreaticoduodenal artery is transected as the dissection continues along the SMA with the Ligasure. After completing a cholecystectomy, the specimen is extracted, and the reconstruction phase is initiated.

Pancreaticojejunostomy
The jejunal limb is brought up to the RUQ through the root of the mesentery as a neo-duodenum and laid comfortably with the antimesenteric border facing the transected pancreatic neck stump. The pancreaticojejunostomy is performed using a modified Blumgart technique (**Fig. 2**D). Three horizontal mattress 3-0 silk sutures are placed, a duct to mucosa anastomoses is performed using 5-0 polydioxanone sutures over a 4- or 5-French stent and finally the 2-0 silks are used to complete the anterior outer layer.

Hepaticojejunostomy
An end-to-side hepaticojejunostomy is performed in a continuous fashion using two 4-0 V-Loc sutures for large ducts (>8 mm, **Fig. 2**E). If the duct is small, then an interrupted anastomosis is performed using 5-0 polydioxanone or 5-0 polyglyconate sutures.

Gastrojejunostomy
An antecolic 2-layer end-to-side hand-sewn isoperistaltic gastrojejunostomy is performed (**Fig. 2**F). Interrupted Lembert 2-0 silk sutures are placed to create the posterior row. A 4 cm segment of the caudal gastric staple line is removed and a corresponding enterotomy is performed using hot scissors. The inner layer of the anastomosis is created using two 3-0 V loc sutures. Finally, the outer layer is completed with interrupted 2-0 silk Lembert sutures.

To conclude the procedure, a 19 French Blake drain is placed posterior to the hepaticojejunostomy and anterior to the pancreaticojejunostomy using the right lateral trocar site. Postoperatively, the patient is managed according to the enhanced recovery pathway.

OUTCOMES OF MINIMALLY INVASIVE PANCREATICODUODENECTOMY

Over the last decade, there has been a steady increase in the use of MIS for pancreaticoduodenectomy, but utilization remains low (under 5%) nationwide because of its complexity.[1] Accompanied with this increased interest is a plethora of reports published on the safety, feasibility, short and long-term oncologic outcomes following this approach. This section will summarize all four published randomized controlled trials and selected national and multi-institutional studies on MIS pancreaticoduodenectomy (**Table 1**).

The PLOT trial was a single-center, open-label, randomized controlled trial performed in India.[17] Sixty-four patients with periampullary cancers were randomized to open versus LPD (32 in each group). The median duration of postoperative hospital stay (13 vs 7 days; $P = .001$) and mean blood loss (250 vs 401 mL; $P<.001$) were lower in the laparoscopy group. The mean duration of the operation was shorter in the open approach (320 vs 359 minutes; $P = .041$). There was no difference in the rates of delayed gastric emptying, pancreatic fistula, postpancreatectomy hemorrhage, overall complication, or mortality.

The PADULAP trial was a single-center open-label randomized controlled trial performed in Spain. Sixty-six patients were randomized to open (n = 32) versus LPD (n = 43).[18] The laparoscopic approach had a shorter median length of stay (13.5 vs17 days; $P = .024$) and longer median operative time (486 vs 365 min; $P = .0001$). The laparoscopic approach had a lower rate of Clavien-Dindo grade $\geq$ 3 complications (5 vs 11 patients; $P = .04$). There were no differences in transfusion requirement, pancreas-specific complications, number of lymph nodes retrieved, and rate of R0 resections between both approaches.

The LEOPARD-2 trial was a multicenter, patient-blinded, parallel-group, randomized controlled phase 2/3 trial performed at four centers in the Netherlands. Patients with benign, premalignant or malignant tumors were randomized to open (n = 49) versus LPD (n = 50). The trial was prematurely terminated by the data and safety monitoring board because of a difference in 90-day complication-related mortality (10% in the laparoscopic group vs 2% in the open approach; $P = .20$). There were no differences in the median time to functional recovery, rate of Clavien-Dindo grade $\geq$ 3 complications and grade B/C POPFs between both groups.

In a more recent multicenter, open-label, randomized controlled trial performed in 14 Chinese medical centers, patients with benign, or malignant pancreatic pathologies were randomized to LPD (n = 328) or OPD (n = 328). The median postoperative length of stay was shorter for patients in the LPD compared with the OPD (15 vs 16 days, $P = .02$). There was no difference in 90-day mortality (2% for both groups) and rate of Clavien-Dindo grade $\geq$ 3 complications (29% for LPD vs 23% for OPD, $P = .13$).

The main limitation of these trials is the use of laparoscopy as the exclusive minimally invasive approach with no trials examining the use of the robot. The DaVinci robotic platform has several potential advantages including wristed instruments, increased dexterity, and 3D vision compared with laparoscopy that may impact critical outcomes of PD including major complications such as pancreatic fistulae. Indeed, several large retrospective analyses not only demonstrate the feasibility and safety of RPD but also indicate advantages over the open and laparoscopic approach.

Table 1
Summary of the randomized trials between minimally invasive pancreatectomy and open approach

Study	Country	Year	Arms	N	Outcomes
PLOT	India	2017	LPD vs OPD	32 vs 32	LPD: • Lower LOS and EBL • Longer operative time • No difference in DGE, POPF, PPH, overall complication or mortality
PADULAP	Spain	2018	LPD vs OPD	34 vs 32	LPD: • Lower LOS and complications • Longer operative time • No difference in transfusion, pancreas-specific complications, number of lymph nodes or R0 resection
LEOPARD-2	Netherlands	2019	LPD vs OPD	50 vs 49	• No difference in median time to function recovery, complications, and POPF • Terminated early because of high 90-d mortality in LPD arm
MITG-P-CPAM trial	China	2021	LPD vs OPD	328 vs 328	LPD: • Lower LOS • No difference in 90-d mortality and serious complications
LEOPARD	Netherlands	2019	MIDP vs ODP	51 vs 57	MIDP: • Lower median time to functional recovery, EBL, and DGE rate • Longer operative time • No difference in complications, POPF, and mortality
LAPOP	Sweden	2020	LDP vs ODP	60 vs 58	LDP: • Lower median time to functional recovery, EBL, and LOS • No difference in complications, DGE, and POPF

Abbreviations: DGE, delayed gastric emptying; EBL, estimated blood loss; LDP, laparoscopic distal pancreatectomy; LOS, length of stay; LPD, laparoscopic pancreaticoduodenectomy; MIDP, minimally invasive distal pancreatectomy; ODP, open distal pancreatectomy; OPD, open pancreatico-duodenectomy; POPF, postoperative pancreatic fistula; PPH, postpancreatectomy hemorrhage.

A multi-institutional study comparing robotic to OPD at 8 high volume centers and surgeons beyond their learning curve for RPD and OPD demonstrated that the robotic approach was associated with longer operative times (mean difference = +75.4 minutes, P = .01) but reduced blood loss (mean difference = −181 minutes, P = .04) compared with OPD. Importantly, RPD was associated with a reduction in major complications (adjusted odds = 0.64, P = .003). There were no differences in 90-day mortality, 90-day readmission, clinically relevant POPF, length of stay, 90-day readmission, or positive resection margin rates.[19] In a large study from the NCDB spanning 7 years (2010–2016), 626 RPDs for PDAC were compared with 17,205 OPDs. The robotic approach was associated with increased rates of adequate lymphadenectomy and a shorter length of stay. There was no difference in 90-day mortality and median overall survival between both groups.[8] In another analysis from the 2014 to 2015 pancreas-targeted American College of Surgeons National Surgical Quality Improvement Program, when compared with the laparoscopic approach, the robotic approach was associated with a lower conversion rate (11.4% vs 26%, P = .041).[10] Conversion has been shown to be associated with an increase in overall complications, length of stay, and likelihood of nonhome discharge.[20]

Collectively, these data indicate that the use of MIS is safe, feasible, and oncologically adequate, especially if used in the appropriately selected patient population and performed by experienced and trained surgeons.

TECHNICAL ASPECTS OF ROBOTIC DISTAL PANCREATECTOMY
Positioning

Similar to RPD, the patient is positioned supine on a split leg table with the legs abducted to allow for the bedside assistant to stand between the legs. In this case, the right arm is placed on an arm board and the left arm is tucked. The patient should be appropriately padded and anchored well to the table with circumferential straps over the chest and legs. The operative table is placed in steep Trendelenburg and the XI robot is docked from the right side of the patient.

Using a 5 mm zero-degree scope and an optical trocar, the abdomen is accessed in the left upper quadrant. The abdomen is insufflated to 15 mm Hg, a diagnostic laparoscopy is performed, and 6 additional ports are placed, as described in **Fig. 1**B.

The Steps of the Operation

Pancreatic exposure
The initial portion of the operation is usually performed laparoscopically. A thin area in the gastrocolic ligament is identified along the mid to distal third of the greater curvature, through which the lesser is accessed. The Ligasure is used to take down the gastrocolic ligament and short gastric vessels up to the angle of His. Medially, the dissection is carried out to the level of the GDA to expose the pancreatic neck. The liver retractor is now placed from the right lateral port and used to retract the stomach and left lateral sector of the liver. The splenic flexure is mobilized, and the robot is docked thereafter from the right side of the patient.

Division of the splenic vessels
The splenic artery is dissected circumferentially at the superior edge of the pancreas using the hook cautery and transected with an endo GIA stapler using 45 mm gold load (**Fig. 3**A). If the coronary veins are encountered, then they can be divided using the Ligasure. Next, the splenic vein is circumferentially dissected at the inferior border of the pancreas and transected with endo GIA stapler using 45 mm gold load (**Fig. 3**B).

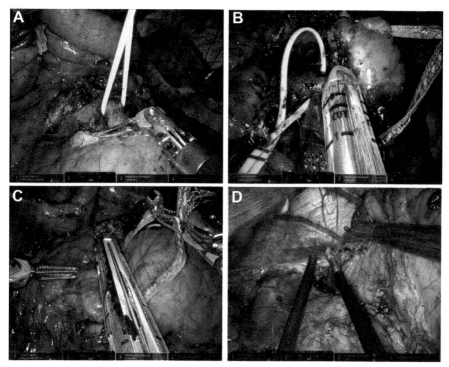

Fig. 3. (*A*) Transection of the splenic artery. (*B*) Transection of the splenic vein, which can be performed before or after pancreas transection. (*C*) Pancreas transection. (*D*) Takedown of retroperitoneal tissue.

Pancreas transection and resection off the retroperitoneum

A tunnel is created under the pancreas and an umbilical tape is used to encircle it. Then the pancreas is transected with an endo GIA stapler using 60 mm purple or black load depending on the thickness of the gland (**Fig. 3C**). Finally, the pancreas is dissected off the retroperitoneum and the spleen is mobilized by dividing all the suspending ligaments (**Fig. 3D**). The specimen is extracted, and a 19-French Blake drain is placed through the left lateral trocar site. Postoperatively, the patient is managed according to the enhanced recovery pathway.

OUTCOMES OF MINIMALLY INVASIVE DISTAL PANCREATECTOMY

Although the adoption of MIS has been slow for pancreaticoduodenectomy, it has been more rigorous for distal pancreatectomy because of a relatively less challenging dissection and the lack of a reconstruction phase. There is a plethora of analyses supporting the adoption of this approach, 2 of which are randomized trials and are presented below.[21–40]

The LEOPARD trial was a multicenter patient-blinded, randomized controlled superiority trial performed in 14 centers of the Dutch Pancreatic Cancer Group. Patients with left-sided pancreatic tumors without vascular involvement were randomized to MIDP (*n* = 51, 42 laparoscopic and 5 robotic) and open distal pancreatectomy (*n* = 57). The median time to functional recovery (4 vs 6 days; *P*<.001) and operative blood loss (150 mL vs 400 mL; *P*<.001) were lower in the MIDP group compared with the ODP group. On the contrary, the median operative time was longer in the MIDP group (217 vs 179 minutes; $P<.001$). There were no differences in Clavien-Dindo grade ≥ 3 complications, POPF grade B/C, percutaneous catheter drainage, or 90-day mortality but there was a decrease in the rate of delayed gastric emptying B/C in the MIDP group (6% vs 20%; $P<.04$). Quality of life was better after MIDP and overall costs were nonsignificantly less after MIDP.

In the second randomized, unblinded, single-center trial performed in Sweden (LAPOP), patients with benign or malignant lesions in the body or tail of the pancreas were randomized to LDP ($n = 29$) or ODP ($n = 29$). The median postoperative hospital stay (5 vs 6 days, $P = .002$), time to functional recovery (4 vs 6 days, $P = .007$), and blood loss (50 vs 100 mL, $P<.018$) were significantly lower in the LPD group. There were no differences in Clavien-Dindo grade ≥ 3 complication rates, delayed gastric emptying, and clinically relevant POPF between both groups.

These encouraging results along with many retrospective analyses favoring the minimally approach were the basis for the recommendation of the Miami International Evidence-Based Guidelines to support the use of minimally invasive approach for distal pancreatectomy.

SUMMARY

Although adoption has been slow, minimally invasive approaches to pancreatic surgery are continuously being evaluated with the aim of reducing perioperative morbidity. For distal pancreatectomy, MIS is becoming the standard of care, especially for benign pathologies and most malignancies. Randomized controlled trials should be able to delineate the advantages—if any—to the robotic platform over standard laparoscopy for DP. For pancreatoduodenectomy, trials of open versus laparoscopic surgery do not show major benefits. The robotic approach holds several theoretical advantages over laparoscopy and open surgery but needs to be evaluated prospectively. Regardless of approach, minimally invasive pancreatectomy is likely to demonstrate benefits over the open approach if performed on select patients by high-volume surgeons trained in both open and minimally invasive pancreatic surgery.

REFERENCES

1. Hoehn RS, Nassour I, Adam MA, et al. National trends in robotic pancreas surgery. J Gastrointest Surg 2020;1–8. https://doi.org/10.1007/s11605-020-04591-w.
2. Boone BA, Zenati M, Hogg ME, et al. Assessment of quality outcomes for robotic pancreaticoduodenectomy: identification of the learning curve. JAMA Surg 2015; 150(5):416–22.
3. Zureikat AH, Beane JD, Zenati MS, et al. 500 minimally invasive robotic pancreatoduodenectomies: one decade of optimizing performance. Ann Surg 2019;1. https://doi.org/10.1097/sla.0000000000003550.
4. Wright GP, Zureikat AH. Development of minimally invasive pancreatic surgery: an evidence-based systematic review of laparoscopic versus robotic approaches. J Gastrointest Surg 2016;20(9):1658–65.
5. Knab LM, Zenati MS, Khodakov A, et al. Evolution of a novel robotic training curriculum in a complex general surgical oncology fellowship. Ann Surg Oncol 2018; 25(12):3445–52.
6. de Rooij T, van Hilst J, Boerma D, et al. Impact of a nationwide training program in minimally invasive distal pancreatectomy (LAELAPS). Ann Surg 2016;264(5): 754–62.

7. Zwart MJW, Nota CLM, de Rooij T, et al. Outcomes of a multicenter training program in robotic pancreatoduodenectomy (LAELAPS-3). Ann Surg 2021. https://doi.org/10.1097/sla.0000000000004783. Publish Ahead of Print.

8. Nassour I, Winters SB, Hoehn R, et al. Long-term oncologic outcomes of robotic and open pancreatectomy in a national cohort of pancreatic adenocarcinoma. J Surg Oncol 2020;122(2):234–42.

9. Nassour I, Wang SC, Christie A, et al. Minimally invasive versus open pancreaticoduodenectomy: a propensity-matched study from a national cohort of patients. Ann Surg 2017;268(1):1.

10. Nassour I, Wang SC, Porembka MR, et al. Robotic versus laparoscopic pancreaticoduodenectomy: a NSQIP analysis. J Gastrointest Surg 2017;21(11):1784–92. https://doi.org/10.1007/s11605-017-3543-6.

11. Nassour I, Choti MA, Porembka MR, et al. Robotic-assisted versus laparoscopic pancreaticoduodenectomy: oncological outcomes. Surg Endosc 2018;32(6): 2907–13.

12. Asbun HJ, Moekotte AL, Vissers FL, et al. The Miami international evidence-based guidelines on minimally invasive pancreas resection. Ann Surg 2020; 271(1):1–14.

13. Wang M, Meng L, Cai Y, et al. Learning curve for laparoscopic pancreaticoduodenectomy: a CUSUM analysis. J Gastrointest Surg 2016;20(5):924–35.

14. Kim S, Yoon Y-S, Han H-S, et al. Evaluation of a single surgeon's learning curve of laparoscopic pancreaticoduodenectomy: risk-adjusted cumulative summation analysis. Surg Endosc 2021;35(6):2870–8.

15. Song KB, Kim SC, Lee W, et al. Laparoscopic pancreaticoduodenectomy for periampullary tumors: lessons learned from 500 consecutive patients in a single center. Surg Endosc 2020;34(3):1343–52.

16. Sharpe SM, Talamonti MS, Wang CE, et al. Early national experience with laparoscopic pancreaticoduodenectomy for ductal adenocarcinoma: a comparison of laparoscopic pancreaticoduodenectomy and open pancreaticoduodenectomy from the national cancer data base. J Am Coll Surg 2015;221(1):175–84.

17. Palanivelu C, Senthilnathan P, Sabnis SC, et al. Randomized clinical trial of laparoscopic versus open pancreatoduodenectomy for periampullary tumours. Br J Surg 2017;104(11):1443–50.

18. Poves I, Burdío F, Morató O, et al. Comparison of perioperative outcomes between laparoscopic and open approach for pancreatoduodenectomy. Ann Surg 2018;268(5):731–9.

19. Zureikat AH, Postlewait LM, Liu Y, et al. A multi-institutional comparison of perioperative outcomes of robotic and open pancreaticoduodenectomy. Ann Surg 2016;264(4):640–9.

20. Hester CA, Nassour I, Christie A, et al. Predictors and outcomes of converted minimally invasive pancreaticoduodenectomy: a propensity score matched analysis. Surg Endosc 2020;34(2):544–50.

21. Butturini G, Damoli I, Crepaz L, et al. A prospective non-randomised single-center study comparing laparoscopic and robotic distal pancreatectomy. Surg Endosc 2015;29(11):1–8.

22. Mehrabi A, Hafezi M, Arvin J, et al. A systematic review and meta-analysis of laparoscopic versus open distal pancreatectomy for benign and malignant lesions of the pancreas: It's time to randomize. Surgery 2015;157(1): 45–55.

23. Magge D, Gooding W, Choudry H, et al. Comparative effectiveness of minimally invasive and open distal pancreatectomy for ductal adenocarcinoma. JAMA Surg 2013;148(6):525–31.
24. Björnsson B, Larsson AL, Hjalmarsson C, et al. Comparison of the duration of hospital stay after laparoscopic or open distal pancreatectomy: randomized controlled trial. Br J Surg 2020;107(10):1281–8.
25. Magge DR, Zenati MS, Hamad A, et al. Comprehensive comparative analysis of cost-effectiveness and perioperative outcomes between open, laparoscopic, and robotic distal pancreatectomy. HPB (Oxford) 2018;20(12):1172–80.
26. Nassour I, Wang SC, Porembka MR, et al. Conversion of minimally invasive distal pancreatectomy: predictors and outcomes. Ann Surg Oncol 2017;24(12): 3725–31.
27. Lee SY, Allen PJ, Sadot E, et al. Distal pancreatectomy: a single institution's experience in open, laparoscopic, and robotic approaches. J Am Coll Surg 2015; 220(1):18–27.
28. Duran H, Ielpo B, Caruso R, et al. Does robotic distal pancreatectomy surgery offer similar results as laparoscopic and open approach? A comparative study from a single medical center. Int J Med Robot 2014;10(3):280–5.
29. Kantor O, Bryan DS, Talamonti MS, et al. Laparoscopic distal pancreatectomy for cancer provides oncologic outcomes and overall survival identical to open distal pancreatectomy. J Gastrointest Surg 2017;21(10):1–6.
30. Bauman MD, Becerra DG, Kilbane EM, et al. Laparoscopic distal pancreatectomy for pancreatic cancer is safe and effective. Surg Endosc 2017;32(1):1–9.
31. Sulpice L, Farges O, Goutte N, et al. Laparoscopic distal pancreatectomy for pancreatic ductal adenocarcinoma. Ann Surg 2015;262(5):868–74.
32. Sahakyan MA, Kim SC, Kleive D, et al. Laparoscopic distal pancreatectomy for pancreatic ductal adenocarcinoma: Long-term oncologic outcomes after standard resection. Surgery 2017;162(4):802–11.
33. Jayaraman S, Gonen M, Brennan MF, et al. Laparoscopic distal pancreatectomy: evolution of a technique at a single institution. J Am Coll Surg 2010;211(4):503–9.
34. Riviere D, Gurusamy KS, Kooby DA, et al. Laparoscopic versus open distal pancreatectomy for pancreatic cancer. GI CU, Group PD. Cochrane Database Syst Rev 2016;29(7):1871–964.
35. Sui C-J, Li B, Yang J-M, et al. Laparoscopic versus open distal pancreatectomy: A meta-analysis. Asian J Surg 2012;35(1):1–8.
36. Adam MA, Choudhury K, Goffredo P, et al. Minimally invasive distal pancreatectomy for cancer: short-term oncologic outcomes in 1733 patients. World J Surg 2015;39(10):2564–72.
37. Raoof M, Nota CLMA, Melstrom LG, et al. Oncologic outcomes after robot-assisted versus laparoscopic distal pancreatectomy: Analysis of the National Cancer Database. J Surg Oncol 2018;118(4):651–6.
38. van Hilst J, Korrel M, de Rooij T, et al. Oncologic outcomes of minimally invasive versus open distal pancreatectomy for pancreatic ductal adenocarcinoma: A systematic review and meta-analysis. Eur J Surg Oncol 2018;45(Ann Surg 255 6 2012):719–27.
39. Raoof M, Ituarte PHG, Woo Y, et al. Propensity score-matched comparison of oncological outcomes between laparoscopic and open distal pancreatic resection. Br J Surg 2018;105(5):578–86.
40. Chopra A, Nassour I, Zureikat A, et al. Perioperative and oncologic outcomes of open, laparoscopic, and robotic distal pancreatectomy for pancreatic adenocarcinoma. Updates Surg 2021;1–7. https://doi.org/10.1007/s13304-020-00927-y.

Health Care Disparities and the Future of Pancreatic Cancer Care

Marianna V. Papageorge, MD[a], Douglas B. Evans, MD[b],
Jennifer F. Tseng, MD, MPH[a],*

KEYWORDS

- Pancreatic cancer • Healthcare disparities • Social determinants of health
- Racial disparities

KEY POINTS

- Pancreatic cancer remains an unsolved health care challenge and disparities in care have been identified in incidence, stage at diagnosis, treatment, and survival based on race, sex, socioeconomic status, and geography.
- The mechanisms underlying these disparities include both patient-specific and health care system–specific factors.
- Future steps to achieve equitable pancreatic cancer care should include improved research methods and comprehensive policy measures to address these disparities.

INTRODUCTION

Pancreatic cancer is the third leading cause of cancer death, with approximately 57,600 new diagnoses and 47,000 deaths expected in the United States in 2020.[1] The mortality of this disease is high, with a 5-year survival of 10%, as the disease is systemic at diagnosis in most patients.[2] Treatment is based on the extent of disease; however, for patients who have a performance status, comorbidity profile, and support system acceptable to receive therapy, current treatment sequencing is largely stage agnostic. All patients receive systemic therapy first (regardless of stage) and subsequent treatments may include surgery and/or radiation therapy.[3] The unique challenge we have in treating patients with pancreatic cancer involves the complexity and potential toxicity of currently available therapies and the multisystem nature of the disease. Biliary obstruction, gastric outlet obstruction, nutritional and intravascular

Conflicts of Interest: No conflicts of interest to disclose. Dr M.V. Papageorge is supported by a T32 grant through Boston University School of Medicine (award #T32HP10028).
^a Boston Medical Center, Boston University School of Medicine, 88 East Newton Street, Collamore - C500, Boston, MA 02118, USA; ^b Department of Surgery, Medical College of Wisconsin, 8701 Watertown Plank Road, Wilwaukee, WI 53226, USA
* Corresponding author.
E-mail address: Jennifer.Tseng@bmc.org
Twitter: @MPapageorge_MD (M.V.P.); @DougEvans2273 (D.B.E.); @TsengJennifer (J.F.T.)

volume depletion, pain, and depression can make successful treatment impossible for many patients. There may be no other solid tumor in which the social determinants of health influence the successful receipt of anticancer therapy more significantly than in patients with pancreatic cancer. Chemotherapy, radiation therapy, and recovery from surgery are difficult to impossible in the absence of social/family support, access to food and transportation, and a basic understanding of the goals of care, to include recognition of the toxicities of treatment. Currently available anticancer therapies for patients with pancreatic cancer are not a realistic goal in patients with significant underlying comorbidities. When comorbidities are combined/added to an environment characterized by inadequacies in many social determinates of health, then (successful) treatment becomes very difficult or impossible; this individual assessment of whether the treatment may be worse than the disease (for a given patient) is made by oncologists/surgeons every day, something that greatly complicates research into the effect of health systems on disparities of pancreatic cancer care. Even when the patient appears physiologically treatable, patient factors included in the social determinants of health may also make successful treatment impossible. As we will describe in this article, disparities in health care that influence patient comorbidities and disparities in social determinants of health confound the analysis of disparities in pancreatic cancer treatment. The goal of anticancer therapy is to maximize length and quality of survival; there are times when a decision in favor of treatment shortens patient survival. When this occurs, it is often due to underlying comorbidities or lack of patient support (as broadly defined). As the disease-associated morbidity and the toxicity of available therapies become greater, the influence of social determinants of health on tolerance and success of treatment becomes more powerful.

To further complicate matters, pancreatic cancer disproportionately affects nonwhite, lower income, and uninsured populations.[4–6] This disparity ultimately translates to worse outcomes for these patients.[7] As mentioned previously, disparities in care and outcomes are complicated, and tied to societal factors such as race and socioeconomic status, which ultimately impact access, treatment, and survival. This article works to outline factors underlying disparities in diagnosis, treatment, and outcomes, and provide recommendations for the future of pancreatic cancer care.

SCOPE OF THE PROBLEM
Incidence

The incidence of pancreatic cancer has been noted to be 50% to 90% higher among black individuals as compared with white individuals in the United States.[8,9] Increased incidence is also seen in male individuals and in those with lower socioeconomic status.[10] These trends have remained largely unchanged over time. It has been argued that these populations are disproportionately affected due to behavioral risk factors, such as smoking and obesity.[11] Although these factors may attribute to an increased incidence, they do not completely explain the disparity.[4]

Stage at Diagnosis

Black patients present more often with advanced-stage disease as compared with white patients.[7,12,13] This is also seen with insurance and socioeconomic status, as the uninsured and those of lower socioeconomic status present at later stages.[6,12]

Treatment

Disparities in surgical resection have been demonstrated based on socioeconomic status, race, marital status, insurance status, and geographic location.[6,12,14,15] Not only are black patients less likely than white patients to undergo evaluation by a surgeon, after adjustment for patient demographics, tumor characteristics, socioeconomic status, and year of diagnosis, these patients were up to 43% less likely to undergo resection for localized cancer once seen by a surgeon.[5,16] This racial disparity is paralleled in chemotherapy, as black patients are less likely to receive adjuvant treatment.[13,16] Similarly, those of lower socioeconomic status are less likely to receive surgical resection, chemotherapy, or radiation.[17] For patients with lower socioeconomic status who do undergo resection, they are less likely to receive the recommended treatment per National Comprehensive Cancer Network guidelines.[18] Adjunct therapies, such as endoscopic retrograde cholangiopancreatography and hospice care, are used less often in nonwhite populations and in certain regions of the country.[19,20] Last, a recent retrospective cohort study of Medicare beneficiaries identified longer wait times between diagnosis and surgical intervention in both female and older patients.[21]

Survival

Historically, the literature has overwhelmingly reported worse outcomes for nonwhite patients and those of lower socioeconomic status.[9,10,16] Multiple studies have demonstrated that black and Hispanic patients have shorter overall survival and higher rates of postoperative complications, in-hospital mortality, and prolonged hospital stay as compared with white patients, even after adjustment for confounders.[14,22–25] More recently, multiple large retrospective studies using state or national cancer databases have found that race is independently associated with worse survival, but this association was no longer significant after controlling for confounders.[13,26,27] These studies highlight the value of stage-appropriate treatment and point to the need for further study of underlying disparities.

When evaluating survival based on socioeconomic status, a retrospective study using the Florida Cancer Registry demonstrated that individuals with lower socioeconomic status, although younger at the time of diagnosis, were not only less likely to undergo appropriate treatment, but overall had higher perioperative and long-term mortality rates, after adjusting for patient comorbidities.[17] Similarly, a retrospective study using a population-based cancer registry in Japan evaluated pancreatic cancer outcomes based on occupational class, as a proxy for socioeconomic status, and found that even in the setting of universal health coverage, higher class occupations had improved cancer survival.[28]

Beyond race and socioeconomic status, access and institutional characteristics, such as volume and location, can result in disparities in outcomes.[6,29–33]

DISCUSSION
Mechanisms Underlying Disparities

To understand the mechanisms underlying disparities in pancreatic cancer, two domains must be evaluated: patient factors and health care system factors. Patient factors include clinical characteristics (risk factors), social demographics (insurance status and socioeconomic status), and preferences and beliefs. Health care system factors include both physician (referrals, communication, and bias) and hospital (volume and location) factors. These two contexts contribute to the utilization and quality of pancreatic cancer care (**Fig. 1**).

Patient Factors

Comorbidities and risk factors
Multiple risk factors have been associated with increased incidence, perioperative complications, and mortality in pancreatic cancer, including obesity, diabetes, and

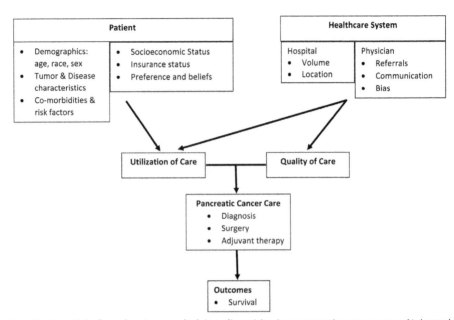

Fig. 1. A model of mechanisms underlying disparities in pancreatic cancer care. (Adapted with permission from Morris AM, et al. Understanding racial disparities in cancer treatment and outcomes. J Am Coll Surg. 2010 Jul;211(1):105-13.)

tobacco use.[3,34,35] A recent retrospective analysis in Georgia found a number of factors to be associated with incidence and mortality in patients with pancreatic cancer, including health behaviors (such as tobacco use, alcohol use, diet, and exercise), economic factors (a composite measure of education, employment, income, and social support) and physical environment (a composite measure of safety and built environment).[11] It must be noted that many of these risk factors occur in higher incidence in poorer, nonwhite populations, reflecting the systemic challenges associated with poor health outcomes and social determinants of health.

Socioeconomic status
Socioeconomic status is an economic and sociologic measure that includes factors such as income, education, and occupation. It has been demonstrated that higher socioeconomic status is associated with increased receipt of treatment, decreased time to treatment, and overall longer survival in patients with pancreatic cancer.[36] Socioeconomic status is often used as a proxy for education, race, and urban environment, but in reality, stands alone in its effect on diagnosis, treatment, and patient outcome.

Insurance status
Uninsured status has been linked to later stage of disease at diagnosis, delayed receipt of treatment, and worse cancer-specific mortality.[6,12,27,37,38] A retrospective cohort study of patients with pancreatic cancer following the Massachusetts health care reform demonstrated that expansion of coverage resulted in increased surgical resection rates.[39] Similarly, a study done within the Department of Defense demonstrated no differences in patient management or survival in black and white patients with pancreatic cancer. This was attributed to the universal access health care system available to these patients.[40]

Other patient factors
Patients' beliefs and preferences may affect their decisions to undergo cancer treatment and thus impact outcomes. For instance, black patients are more likely to be documented as refusing surgery for pancreatic cancer.[27,41] This could represent suboptimal communication by providers, mistrust in the context of historical medical exploitation, or other factors influencing patient choice.[42]

Physician Factors

Referrals
Undertreatment of patients with pancreatic cancer may also be a result of a decreased rate of referrals. This has been documented in large US database studies, in which black patients were less likely to be referred to a medical oncologist, radiation oncologist, or surgeon.[14,16] Similarly, in a retrospective analysis in Australia, rural residence was associated with decreased referral to a medical oncologist for individuals with advanced pancreatic cancer.[43] This may be partially explained by the pessimistic outlook that many nonspecialty physicians may have regarding treatment success for this disease. Outside of the United States and parts of Europe, there exists a fatalistic attitude on the part of many physicians, especially those with a broad practice in family medicine.

Patient-physician communication
Effective communication, which includes factors such as empathy, physician attentiveness, and shared decision making, can affect patient quality of life, satisfaction with care, and medical outcomes in oncology.[44–47] For example, in a prospective cohort study of patients diagnosed with early-stage lung cancer, negative perceptions of patient-physician communication were significantly associated with decisions against surgery.[48]

Effective communication must also be sensitive to a patient's primary language and health literacy. Language has been studied less extensively in cancer outcomes as compared with other social determinants of health, and published data have demonstrated mixed results with regard to disparities in outcomes. There is a clear difference in patients' reports and ratings of care, as non-English speakers report worse care as compared with English speakers.[49–54] Similarly, poor health literacy has been tied to poor overall health outcomes, along with cancer care.[55,56] Patients with poor health literacy may have misconceptions about their care and ineffective communication with their provider, leading to suboptimal treatment, poor adherence to treatment recommendations, or dissatisfaction.

Bias
Both implicit and explicit bias can affect physicians' perceptions of patients and treatment options. Race, socioeconomic status, and gender have been negatively associated with physicians' assessment of patient intelligence and personality, as well as risk behavior and the likelihood of adhering to treatment recommendations.[57–59] This bias not only results in inequitable outcomes but can undermine the physician-patient relationship. It is important to note that all providers suffer from some form of implicit bias, but the examination of these biases can lead to improved care and outcomes.[60]

Hospital Factors

Volume
Hospital volume is a well-established measure of quality in cancer care.[61] Multiple studies have demonstrated that higher-volume centers and higher-volume surgeons are associated with improved outcomes in pancreatic cancer care.[30,33,62,63] A retrospective cohort study using the National Inpatient Sample demonstrated that 38.2%

of pancreatic resections were performed at high-volume centers. Of these, nonwhite patients, those with a greater number of comorbidities, and those in lower income groups were more likely to have their surgery performed at a low-volume hospital.[64] A retrospective cohort study using data from New York City demonstrated similar findings, in which nonwhite patients were significantly less likely to be treated at high-volume hospitals and/or with a high-volume surgeon.[65] The reasoning for this disparity is not clear, but may represent inequitable access and resource distribution. As the wave of physician employment continues across this country, narrow network insurance plans will impede access to high-volume centers and potentially further restrict access to care.

Location
The location of cancer care, including region, distance, and urban versus rural environment, has been demonstrated to impact outcomes in patients with pancreatic care. Patients from rural areas were more likely to present with later-stage disease and had an increased risk of death compared with patients from urban areas.[66,67] Interestingly, two recent studies evaluated the treatment and outcomes at urban, safety-net hospitals and found no significant differences based on social determinants of health, demonstrating that these hospitals may be well-equipped to provide equitable outcomes for disproportionately low-income, less-educated, and less-white populations.[68,69] Multiple studies have demonstrated regional and geographic variations in treatment and outcomes.[12,15,70] The true cause of these disparities may reflect a combination of factors, including access, source and quality of care, clinical recommendations, and patient preference.

FUTURE DIRECTIONS

Pancreatic cancer incidence continues to increase, and in the next two years, it is predicted that pancreatic cancer will be the second leading cause of cancer death in the United States.[71] To address disparities in diagnosis, treatment, and outcomes, targeted improvements are called for in research, policy, and clinical care.

Research

Improved data collection
To better understand pancreatic cancer disparities, more precise data collection is required. With regard to race, methods for collecting data include extraction, proxy report, and direct observation and self-report. Of these, self-report is the optimal method and should be used when feasible.

With regard to socioeconomic status, the use of individual-level income is not reliable and thus census tract or zip code level should be used as estimation.[72] As previously noted, some have argued for the use of socioeconomic status as a proxy for race, education, and urban environment, but this is not ideal. These relationships are not reciprocal, and given the history of systemic racism in the United States, the effects of race on health are multifactorial, of which only part is socioeconomic status, education, and environment.

Last, not only are more precise definitions required, but more focused research on barriers to utilization and high-quality care is required to understand and address the mechanisms underlying disparities.

Research methodologies
Due to the multilevel factors affecting disparities, including patient, provider, institution, and region, a hierarchical modeling approach may be more helpful than

traditional regression techniques. In addition, techniques such as qualitative research and community-based participatory research may be a better tool to understand gaps in care and provide population-specific interventions.[73]

Risk adjustment

Risk-adjustment and prediction models often rely on aggregated datasets. As previously noted, such data collection can be flawed and these models can often perpetuate race-based health inequities. This has been seen recently with the reevaluation of the use of race in glomerular filtration rate, which has resulted in racial disparities in dialysis and kidney transplantation.[74] This is one example of many in which prediction models require reevaluation.

Policy

Access

As discussed previously, insurance status is a significant contributor to pancreatic cancer disparities. Expansion of insurance availability, for example, through the Medicaid expansion of the Affordable Care Act, has demonstrated improvements in screening, earlier-stage diagnoses, and surgical access in certain cancer types.[75] These gains were also highlighted in nonwhite and previously uninsured populations. Therefore, the expansion of accessible care should be prioritized, as it will likely benefit patients with pancreatic cancer and those for whom disparities exist.

Patient-centered tools

The first patient navigator program was created in 1990 in response to poor access to and follow-up of breast cancer screening in Harlem.[76] Since that time, use of this intervention, focused on coordination, communication, and addressing barriers to care, has increased and has been shown to improve screening rates and timely follow-up care.[77] The National Cancer Institute has initiated a Patient Navigation Research Program to evaluate timely screening and care, along with patient satisfaction and cost-effectiveness for breast, cervical, colon, and prostate cancer.[78] This research effort is an important first step in the understanding of the widespread use of patient navigators in cancer care.

Hospital incentives and quality measures

Value-based incentive programs for hospital reimbursement have gained significant traction in the past two decades and are a core tenant of Medicare reimbursement. The goal of these programs is to provide high-quality care, resulting in improved health and lower costs. Often, these incentive systems do not include decreased racial disparities as a target.[79] In fact, providers and hospitals that serve nonwhite patients and patients of lower socioeconomic status often have lower quality-of-care measures.[80–82] Under the current models, these lower scores can result in decreased payments and potentially worsening health care disparities. Therefore, this must be taken into consideration when creating payment models and disparity reduction must be included as a quality improvement measure.

Diversity in physician workforce

Studies suggest that racial and gender concordance can enhance patient experience and physician communication.[83] This is critical to understand when evaluating the makeup of the present-day physician workforce. With regard to gender, women make up 50% of present-day medical school classes but only 35% of practicing physicians.[84] In addition, there remain clear disparities in surgical subspecialties and positions of leadership.[85,86] With regard to race, only 5% of practicing physicians identify as black as compared with 56% who identify as white.[87] This disparity in black physicians has remained largely unchanged over time.[88] Last, with regard to socioeconomic status, one-third of the US population lives at or near the poverty line, whereas only 7% of medical students come from these backgrounds.[89] The average student graduates from medical school with more than $200,000 in debt, with only 14% of students graduating without loans.[90] To create a physician workforce that treats a diverse group of patients, enhanced support systems are required to attract and attain physicians of all backgrounds and to encourage them to work in safety-net systems/hospitals.

Combating structural racism and systemic oppression

The disparities outlined previously are multifactorial and cannot be discussed without attributing their origins to a history of structural racism and systemic oppression, particularly among nonwhite and lower socioeconomic status individuals. For example, in areas of higher segregation, often a result of red-lining and housing discrimination, black patients with pancreatic cancer were more likely to present with advanced-stage disease, less likely to receive the appropriate surgical care, and had overall worse survival as compared with white patients.[91] These differences disappear in areas of higher integration between black and white patients. Future efforts in medicine and beyond must prioritize policies and funding to combat these systems of oppression and support these populations in need.

SUMMARY

Pancreatic cancer will represent one of the major health care challenges of the next decade (and beyond); our failure to achieve equitable outcomes for all patient populations must be addressed. These disparities in incidence, management, and outcomes can be broadly thought of as due to both patient and health care system factors. To ensure that all patient populations receive appropriate treatment and optimal outcomes, we must put in place targeted measures to address gaps in research, access, patient needs, hospital factors, and systemic models. Only through these efforts will the causes of such inequitable outcomes be understood and strategies developed to minimize disparities in pancreatic cancer care.

CLINICS CARE POINTS

- Disparities in pancreatic cancer care have been identified in incidence, stage at diagnosis, treatment, and survival based on race, sex, socioeconomic status, and geography.

- The mechanisms underlying these disparities can be evaluated on both a patient and health care system level. Patient-specific factors include clinical characteristics (risk factors), social demographics (insurance status and socioeconomic status), and preferences and beliefs. Health care system factors include physician (referrals, communication, and bias) and hospital factors (volume and location).

- Future steps in pancreatic cancer care should address research and policy. Improvements in research methods should include collection, methodology, and risk. Policy measures should include expanded access, availability of patient-centered tools, hospital incentives, and quality measures based on decreasing disparities, increased workforce diversity, and combating systemic oppression.

REFERENCES

1. Pancreatic Cancer: Statistics. Available at: https://www.cancer.net/cancer-types/pancreatic-cancer/statistics. Accessed December 03, 2020.

2. Cancer Stat Facts: Pancreatic Cancer. 2020. Available at: https://seer.cancer. gov/statfacts/html/pancreas.html. Accessed December 03, 2020.

3. Wolff RA, Crane CH, Li D, et al. Neoplasms of the exocrine pancreas. In Bast RC, Croce CM, Hait WN, et al, eds Holland-Frei Cancer Medicine, 10th edition. Hoboken, NJ: Wiley Blackwell;2017.

4. Khawja SN, Mohammed S, Silberfein EJ, et al. Pancreatic cancer disparities in African Americans. Pancreas 2015;44(4):522–7.

5. Riall TS, Townsend CM Jr, Kuo YF, et al. Dissecting racial disparities in the treatment of patients with locoregional pancreatic cancer: a 2-step process. Cancer 2010;116(4):930–9.

6. Smith JK, Ng SC, Zhou Z, et al. Does increasing insurance improve outcomes for US cancer patients? J Surg Res 2013;185(1):15–20.

7. Noel M, Fiscella K. Disparities in pancreatic cancer treatment and outcomes. Health Equity 2019;3(1):532–40.

8. Silverman DT, Hoover RN, Brown LM, et al. Why do Black Americans have a higher risk of pancreatic cancer than White Americans? Epidemiology (Cambridge, Mass) 2003;14(1):45–54.

9. Vick AD, Hery DN, Markowiak SF, et al. Closing the disparity in pancreatic cancer outcomes: a closer look at nonmodifiable factors and their potential use in treatment. Pancreas 2019;48(2):242–9.

10. Sun H, Ma H, Hong G, et al. Survival improvement in patients with pancreatic cancer by decade: a period analysis of the SEER database, 1981-2010. Sci Rep 2014;4:6747.

11. Brotherton L, Welton M, Robb SW. Racial disparities of pancreatic cancer in Georgia: a county-wide comparison of incidence and mortality across the state, 2000-2011. Cancer Med 2016;5(1):100–10.

12. Shapiro M, Chen Q, Huang Q, et al. Associations of socioeconomic variables with resection, stage, and survival in patients with early-stage pancreatic cancer. JAMA Surg 2016;151(4):338–45.

13. Heller DR, Nicolson NG, Ahuja N, et al. Association of treatment inequity and ancestry with pancreatic ductal adenocarcinoma survival. JAMA Surg 2020; 155(2):e195047.

14. Murphy MM, Simons JP, Hill JS, et al. Pancreatic resection. Cancer 2009;115(17): 3979–90.

15. Kasumova GG, Eskander MF, de Geus SWL, et al. Regional variation in the treatment of pancreatic adenocarcinoma: decreasing disparities with multimodality therapy. Surgery 2017;162(2):275–84.

16. Murphy MM, Simons JP, Ng SC, et al. Racial differences in cancer specialist consultation, treatment, and outcomes for locoregional pancreatic adenocarcinoma. Ann Surg Oncol 2009;16(11):2968–77.

17. Cheung MC, Yang R, Byrne MM, et al. Are patients of low socioeconomic status receiving suboptimal management for pancreatic adenocarcinoma? Cancer 2010;116(3):723–33.

18. Visser BC, Ma Y, Zak Y, et al. Failure to comply with NCCN guidelines for the management of pancreatic cancer compromises outcomes. HPB (Oxford) 2012; 14(8):539–47.

19. Tavakkoli A, Singal AG, Waljee AK, et al. Regional and racial variations in the utilization of endoscopic retrograde cholangiopancreatography among pancreatic cancer patients in the United States. Cancer Med 2019;8(7):3420–7.

20. Paredes AZ, Hyer JM, Palmer E, et al. Racial/ethnic disparities in hospice utilization among medicare beneficiaries dying from pancreatic cancer. J Gastrointest Surg 2020;25(1):155–61.

21. Azap RA, Hyer JM, Diaz A, et al. Sex-based differences in time to surgical care among pancreatic cancer patients: a national study of Medicare beneficiaries. J Surg Oncol 2020;123(1):236–44.

22. Wray CJ, Castro-Echeverry E, Silberfein EJ, et al. A multi-institutional study of pancreatic cancer in Harris County, Texas: race predicts treatment and survival. Ann Surg Oncol 2012;19(9):2776–81.

23. Nipp R, Tramontano AC, Kong CY, et al. Disparities in cancer outcomes across age, sex, and race/ethnicity among patients with pancreatic cancer. Cancer Med 2018;7(2):525–35.

24. Sukumar S, Ravi P, Sood A, et al. Racial disparities in operative outcomes after major cancer surgery in the United States. World J Surg 2015;39(3):634–43.

25. Lucas FL, Stukel TA, Morris AM, et al. Race and surgical mortality in the United States. Ann Surg 2006;243(2):281–6.

26. Zell JA, Rhee JM, Ziogas A, et al. Race, socioeconomic status, treatment, and survival time among pancreatic cancer cases in California. Cancer Epidemiol biomarkers Prev 2007;16(3):546–52.

27. Moaven O, Richman JS, Reddy S, et al. Healthcare disparities in outcomes of patients with resectable pancreatic cancer. Am J Surg 2019;217(4):725–31.

28. Zaitsu M, Kim Y, Lee HE, et al. Occupational class differences in pancreatic cancer survival: A population-based cancer registry-based study in Japan. Cancer Med 2019;8(6):3261–8.

29. Makar M, Worple E, Dove J, et al. Disparities in care: impact of socioeconomic factors on pancreatic surgery: exploring the National Cancer Database. Am Surg 2019;85(4):327–34.

30. McPhee JT, Hill JS, Whalen GF, et al. Perioperative mortality for pancreatectomy: a national perspective. Ann Surg 2007;246(2):246–53.

31. Simons JP, Shah SA, Ng SC, et al. National complication rates after pancreatectomy: beyond mere mortality. J Gastrointest Surg 2009;13(10):1798–805.

32. Chau Z, West JK, Zhou Z, et al. Rankings versus reality in pancreatic cancer surgery: a real-world comparison. HPB (Oxford) 2014;16(6):528–33.

33. Bliss LA, Yang CJ, Chau Z, et al. Patient selection and the volume effect in pancreatic surgery: unequal benefits? HPB (Oxford) 2014;16(10):899–906.

34. Chang EH, Sugiyama G, Smith MC, et al. Obesity and surgical complications of pancreaticoduodenectomy: an observation study utilizing ACS NSQIP. Am J Surg 2020;220(1):135–9.

35. Arnold LD, Patel AV, Yan Y, et al. Are racial disparities in pancreatic cancer explained by smoking and overweight/obesity? Cancer Epidemiol biomarkers Prev 2009;18(9):2397–405.

36. Zhu F, Wang H, Ashamalla H. Racial and socioeconomic disparities in the treatments and outcomes of pancreatic cancer among different treatment facility types. Pancreas 2020;49(10):1355–63.

37. Cole AP, Lu C, Krimphove MJ, et al. Comparing the association between insurance and mortality in ovarian, pancreatic, lung, colorectal, prostate, and breast cancers. J Natl Compr Cancer Netw 2019;17(9):1049–58.

38. Eskander MF, Bliss LA, McCarthy EP, et al. Massachusetts healthcare reform and trends in emergent colon resection. Dis colon rectum 2016;59(11):1063–72.

39. Loehrer AP, Chang DC, Hutter MM, et al. Health insurance expansion and treatment of pancreatic cancer: does increased access lead to improved care? J Am Coll Surg 2015;221(6):1015–22.

40. Lee S, Reha JL, Tzeng CW, et al. Race does not impact pancreatic cancer treatment and survival in an equal access federal health care system. Ann Surg Oncol 2013;20(13):4073–9.

41. Tohme S, Kaltenmeier C, Bou-Samra P, et al. Race and health disparities in patient refusal of surgery for early-stage pancreatic cancer: an NCDB cohort study. Ann Surg Oncol 2018;25(12):3427–35.

42. Byrd WM, Clayton LA. Race, medicine, and health care in the United States: a historical survey. J Natl Med Assoc 2001;93(3 Suppl):11S–34S.

43. Dumbrava MI, Burmeister EA, Wyld D, et al. Chemotherapy in patients with unresected pancreatic cancer in Australia: a population-based study of uptake and survival. Asia Pac J Clin Oncol 2018;14(4):326–36.

44. Baile WF, Aaron J. Patient-physician communication in oncology: past, present, and future. Curr Opin Oncol 2005;17(4):331–5.

45. D'Angelica M, Hirsch K, Ross H, et al. Surgeon-patient communication in the treatment of pancreatic cancer. Arch Surg 1998;133(9):962–6.

46. Zachariae R, Pedersen CG, Jensen AB, et al. Association of perceived physician communication style with patient satisfaction, distress, cancer-related self-efficacy, and perceived control over the disease. Br J Cancer 2003;88(5):658–65.

47. Geessink NH, Ofstad EH, Olde Rikkert MGM, et al. Shared decision-making in older patients with colorectal or pancreatic cancer: determinants of patients' and observers' perceptions. Patient Educ Couns 2018;101(10):1767–74.

48. Cykert S, Dilworth-Anderson P, Monroe MH, et al. Factors associated with decisions to undergo surgery among patients with newly diagnosed early-stage lung cancer. JAMA 2010;303(23):2368–76.

49. Ngai KM, Grudzen CR, Lee R, et al. The association between limited English proficiency and unplanned emergency department revisit within 72 hours. Ann Emerg Med 2016;68(2):213–21.

50. Sarver J, Baker DW. Effect of language barriers on follow-up appointments after an emergency department visit. J Gen Intern Med 2000;15(4):256–64.

51. Carrasquillo O, Orav EJ, Brennan TA, et al. Impact of language barriers on patient satisfaction in an emergency department. J Gen Intern Med 1999;14(2):82–7.

52. Ayanian JZ, Zaslavsky AM, Arora NK, et al. Patients' experiences with care for lung cancer and colorectal cancer: findings from the Cancer Care Outcomes Research and Surveillance Consortium. J Clin Oncol 2010;28(27):4154–61.

53. Feeney T, Cassidy M, Tripodis Y, et al. Association of primary language with outcomes after operations typically performed to treat cancer: analysis of a statewide database. Ann Surg Oncol 2019;26(9):2684–93.

54. Feeney T, Park C, Godley F, et al. Provider–patient language discordance and cancer operations: outcomes from a single center linked to a state vital statistics registry. World J Surg 2020;44(10):3324–32.

55. Koay K, Schofield P, Jefford M. Importance of health literacy in oncology. Asia Pac J Clin Oncol 2012;8(1):14–23.

56. Davis TC, Williams MV, Marin E, et al. Health literacy and cancer communication. CA Cancer J Clin 2002;52(3):134–49.

57. van Ryn M, Burke J. The effect of patient race and socio-economic status on physicians' perceptions of patients. Social Sci Med (1982) 2000;50(6):813–28.

58. Fasano HT, McCarter MSJ, Simonis JM, et al. Influence of socioeconomic bias on emergency medicine resident decision making and patient care. Simul Healthc 2020;16(2):85–91.

59. McIntyre RS, Chen VC, Lee Y, et al. The influence of prescriber and patient gender on the prescription of benzodiazepines: evidence for stereotypes and biases? Social Psychiatry Psychiatr Epidemiol 2020;56(6):1083–9.

60. Kokas M, Fakhoury JW, Hoffert M, et al. Health care disparities: a practical approach to teach residents about self-bias and patient communication. J Racial Ethnic Health Disparities 2019;6(5):1030–4.

61. Birkmeyer JD, Sun Y, Wong SL, et al. Hospital volume and late survival after cancer surgery. Ann Surg 2007;245(5):777–83.

62. Bateni SB, Gingrich AA, Hoch JS, et al. Defining value for pancreatic surgery in early-stage pancreatic cancer. JAMA Surg 2019;154(10):e193019.

63. Eppsteiner RW, Csikesz NG, McPhee JT, et al. Surgeon volume impacts hospital mortality for pancreatic resection. Ann Surg 2009;249(4):635–40.

64. Al-Refaie WB, Muluneh B, Zhong W, et al. Who receives their complex cancer surgery at low-volume hospitals? J Am Coll Surg 2012;214(1):81–7.

65. Epstein AJ, Gray BH, Schlesinger M. Racial and ethnic differences in the use of high-volume hospitals and surgeons. Arch Surg 2010;145(2):179–86.

66. Segel JE, Hollenbeak CS, Gusani NJ. Rural-urban disparities in pancreatic cancer stage of diagnosis: understanding the interaction with medically underserved areas. J Rural Health 2020;36(4):476–83.

67. Markossian TW, O'Neal CM, Senkowski C. Geographic disparities in pancreatic cancer survival in a southeastern safety-net academic medical center. Aust J Rural Health 2016;24(2):73–8.

68. Sridhar P, Misir P, Kwak H, et al. Impact of race, insurance status, and primary language on presentation, treatment, and outcomes of patients with pancreatic adenocarcinoma at a safety-net hospital. J Am Coll Surg 2019;229(4):389–96.

69. Dhar VK, Hoehn RS, Kim Y, et al. Equivalent treatment and survival after resection of pancreatic cancer at safety-net hospitals. J Gastrointest Surg 2018;22(1):98–106.

70. Salami A, Alvarez NH, Joshi ART. Geographic disparities in surgical treatment recommendation patterns and survival for pancreatic adenocarcinoma. HPB (Oxford) 2017;19(11):1008–15.

71. Shah A, Chao KS, Ostbye T, et al. Trends in racial disparities in pancreatic cancer surgery. J Gastrointest Surg 2013;17(11):1897–906.

72. Greenwald HP, Polissar NL, Borgatta EF, et al. Detecting survival effects of socioeconomic status: problems in the use of aggregate measures. J Clin Epidemiol 1994;47(8):903–9.

73. Morris AM, Rhoads KF, Stain SC, et al. Understanding racial disparities in cancer treatment and outcomes. J Am Coll Surg 2010;211(1):105–13.

74. Vyas DA, Eisenstein LG, Jones DS. Hidden in plain sight — reconsidering the use of race correction in clinical algorithms. N Engl J Med 2020;383(9):874–82.

75. Eguia E, Cobb AN, Kothari AN, et al. Impact of the Affordable Care Act (ACA) Medicaid expansion on cancer admissions and surgeries. Ann Surg 2018;268(4):584–90.

76. Freeman HP, Muth BJ, Kerner JF. Expanding access to cancer screening and clinical follow-up among the medically underserved. Cancer Pract 1995;3(1):19–30.

77. Wells KJ, Battaglia TA, Dudley DJ, et al. Patient navigation: state of the art or is it science? Cancer 2008;113(8):1999–2010.

78. Freund KM, Battaglia TA, Calhoun E, et al. National Cancer Institute Patient Navigation Research Program: methods, protocol, and measures. Cancer 2008; 113(12):3391–9.
79. Solving disparities through payment and delivery system reform: a program to achieve health equity. Health Aff 2017;36(6):1133–9.
80. Khullar D, Schpero WL, Bond AM, et al. Association between patient social risk and physician performance scores in the first year of the merit-based incentive payment system. JAMA 2020;324(10):975–83.
81. Sarkar RR, Courtney PT, Bachand K, et al. Quality of care at safety-net hospitals and the impact on pay-for-performance reimbursement. Cancer 2020;126(20): 4584–92.
82. Hsu HE, Wang R, Broadwell C, et al. Association between federal value-based incentive programs and health care–associated infection rates in safety-net and non–safety-net hospitals. JAMA Netw Open 2020;3(7):e209700.
83. Takeshita J, Wang S, Loren AW, et al. Association of racial/ethnic and gender concordance between patients and physicians with patient experience ratings. JAMA Netw Open 2020;3(11):e2024583.
84. Active Physicians by Sex and Speciality, 2017. Available at: https://www.aamc. org/data-reports/workforce/interactive-data/active-physicians-sex-and-specialty-2017. Accessed December 22, 2020.
85. Jena AB, Khullar D, Ho O, et al. Sex differences in academic rank in US medical schools in 2014. JAMA 2015;314(11):1149–58.
86. Zhuge Y, Kaufman J, Simeone DM, et al. Is there still a glass ceiling for women in academic surgery? Ann Surg 2011;253(4):637–43.
87. Diversity in Medicine: Facts and Figures 2019. Available at: https://www.aamc.org/data-reports/workforce/interactive-data/figure-18-percentage-all-active-physicians-race/ethnicity-2018. Accessed December 22, 2020.
88. Laurencin CT, Murray M. An American crisis: the lack of black men in medicine. J Racial Ethnic Health Disparities 2017;4(3):317–21.
89. Baugh AD, Vanderbilt AA, Baugh RF. The dynamics of poverty, educational attainment, and the children of the disadvantaged entering medical school. Adv Med Educ Pract 2019;10:667–76.
90. Craft JA 3rd, Craft TP. Rising medical education debt a mounting concern. Graduates also face less favorable repayment terms, shortage of training positions. Mo Med 2012;109(4):266–70.
91. Blanco BA, Poulson M, Kenzik KM, et al. The impact of residential segregation on pancreatic cancer diagnosis, treatment, and mortality. Ann Surg Oncol 2020; 28(6):3147–55.

Inherited Pancreatic Cancer Syndromes and High-Risk Screening

Leah H. Biller, MD[a], Brian M. Wolpin, MD, MPH[a],*,
Michael Goggins, MB, MD[b],*

KEYWORDS

- Hereditary • Cancer risk • Pancreatic cyst • Surveillance

KEY POINTS

- Individuals with inherited pancreatic cancer predisposition syndromes (both owing to germline pathogenic alterations and family history of pancreatic cancer) may benefit from pancreatic cancer surveillance with endoscopic ultrasound examination and MRI.
- The goal of surveillance is to identify and intervene on high-risk precursor lesions or early-stage cancers.
- Annual pancreatic surveillance results in down-staging of pancreatic cancers that are detected.

INTRODUCTION

In 2020, there will be an estimated 57,600 new cases and 47,050 deaths from pancreatic ductal adenocarcinoma (PDAC) in the United States.[1] With a 5-year survival rate of 9%, PDAC remains a highly lethal disease and often is diagnosed at an advanced, incurable stage.[2] Despite this circumstance, routine surveillance of the general population is not recommended owing to the low incidence and lack of evidence for clinical benefit in asymptomatic individuals.[3]

Although the lifetime risk for developing PDAC in the general population is only 1.6%,[2] a subset of individuals is at increased risk based on inheritance of a germline pathogenic mutation and/or presence of familial PDAC (FPC), defined as families with at least 2 first-degree relatives (FDR) with PDAC without known genetic cause. An underlying hereditary susceptibility is identified in up to 10% of patients with pancreatic adenocarcinoma,[4–9] and professional society guidelines now recommend universal

ª Department of Medical Oncology, Dana-Farber Cancer Institute and Harvard Medical School, 450 Brookline Avenue, Boston, MA, USA; ᵇ Johns Hopkins University, 1550 Orleans Street, Baltimore, MD, USA
* Corresponding authors.
E-mail addresses: brian_wolpin@dfci.harvard.edu (B.M.W.); mgoggins@jhmi.edu (M.G.)
Twitter: @leahbillermd (L.H.B.); @mggoggins (M.G.)

Surg Oncol Clin N Am 30 (2021) 773–786
https://doi.org/10.1016/j.soc.2021.06.002
1055-3207/21/© 2021 Elsevier Inc. All rights reserved.

surgonc.theclinics.com

germline testing for all patients diagnosed with PDAC regardless of family history or age at cancer diagnosis.[10] Although testing may have implications for the proband's cancer treatment, such as with poly (ADP-ribose) polymerase (PARP) inhibitors for BRCA1 or BRCA2 mutation carriers[11] or anti–programmed cell death 1 antibodies for those with Lynch syndrome,[12] results may also risk stratify relatives via cascade testing, which entails testing for the known pathogenic mutation in at-risk family members.

Individuals with inherited PDAC syndromes may benefit from surveillance with cross-sectional imaging studies or endoscopic ultrasound (EUS) examination. The goal of routine screening of high-risk individuals is to improve cancer-associated survival by detecting and intervening early on noninvasive precursor lesions or early-stage cancers. This review discusses the known inherited PDAC syndromes, goals, and methods of screening, as well as surveillance outcomes among high-risk individuals.

INHERITED PANCREATIC DUCTAL ADENOCARCINOMA SYNDROMES
Hereditary Pancreatitis

Hereditary pancreatitis (HP) is a rare syndrome of acute recurrent pancreatitis that frequently leads to the development of chronic pancreatitis by young adulthood. HP is most commonly inherited in an autosomal-dominant fashion owing to pathogenic alterations in PRSS1 (cationic trypsinogen) (**Table 1**). Other genes that have been identified in families with hereditary or familial pancreatitis include SPINK1, CTRC, CFTR, CPA1, and CPB1. PRSS1 mutation carriers have a high penetrance of both pancreatitis and PDAC,[13] although a recent study found that only 7.2% of PRSS1 mutation carriers (83% of whom had pancreatitis) developed PDAC by age 70.[14] Age at diagnosis may depend on time from first clinical episode of pancreatitis[13] and history of cigarette smoking, with ever smokers more likely to develop PDAC, and doing so at a median of 20 years earlier than never smokers.[15]

Long-standing pancreatitis is considered required for the subsequent development of PDAC in mutation carriers, although it may not be always symptomatic. In fact, a recent study of patients with PDAC and deleterious CPA1 and CPB1 variants demonstrated that many patients did not have a prior history of symptomatic pancreatitis.[16] Currently, it is recommended to test for the presence of pancreatitis risk variants only in probands with a clinical and family history suggestive of HP as the population prevalence of HP is only 0.3 per 100,000 (with 68% of cases owing to PRSS1 alterations).[17]

Peutz–Jeghers Syndrome

Peutz–Jeghers syndrome (PJS) is an autosomal-dominant hamartomatous polyposis syndrome most commonly arising in the setting of pathogenic alterations in the STK11/LKB1 gene, a tumor suppressor gene involved in multiple processes related to metabolic regulation. The clinical diagnosis requires 2 of these 3 criteria: at least 2 hamartomas in the gastrointestinal tract; mucocutaneous hyperpigmentation; and/or a family history of PJS.

Patients with PJS are at increased risk of multiple gastrointestinal cancers (including colorectal, stomach, small intestine, and pancreas), as well as female breast, gynecologic, testicular, and lung cancers. A systematic review reported an overall lifetime risk of any cancer of 37% to 93% with a mean age at diagnosis of 42 years.[18] One large study found the cumulative risk of PDAC to be 3%, 5%, 7%, and 11% at ages 40, 50, 60, and 70 years, respectively,[19] although a meta-analysis of 6 studies calculated

Table 1
Inherited PDAC syndromes associated with increased PDAC risk

Syndrome	Gene Name	Lifetime Risk for Pancreatic Cancer	Genetic Mutation Frequency in Pancreatic Cancer Cohorts	Screening Recommendations[a]
HP	PRSS1	7%–40%[13,14]	<0.1	Start at age 40 y or 20 y after developing pancreatitis
Peutz–Jeghers syndrome	STK11	11%–36%[19,20]	<0.1	Start at age 30–35 y or 10 y younger than the earliest diagnosis in the family
Familial atypical mole and multiple melanoma syndrome	CDK2NA	17%[22]	0.3%–0.7%[5,8,9,24]	Start at age 40 y or 10 y younger than the earliest diagnosis in the family
Hereditary breast and ovarian cancer	BRCA1 BRCA2	3%[78] 5%–10%[30]	0.3%–1.3%[5,8,9,31] 1.3%–3.6%[5,8,9,31]	If ≥1 FDR or SDR with PDAC, start at age 50 y or 10 y younger than the earliest diagnosis in the family
Lynch syndrome	MLH1, MSH2, MSH6	4%[36]	1.3%–3.6%[5,8,9,31]	If ≥1 FDR or SDR with PDAC, start at age 50 y or 10 y younger than the earliest diagnosis in the family
Ataxia telangiectasia	ATM	Unknown	1.2%–3.3%[5,6,8,9]	If ≥1 FDR or SDR with PDAC, start at age 50 y or 10 y younger than the earliest diagnosis in the family
Other	PALB2	2%–3%[43]	0.2%–0.4%[5,6,8,9]	If ≥1 FDR or SDR with PDAC, start at age 50 y or 10 y younger than the earliest diagnosis in the family
Li-Fraumeni syndrome	TP53	Unknown	0.12%–0.5%.[5–7]	If ≥1 FDR or SDR with PDAC, start at age 50 y or 10 y younger than the earliest diagnosis in the family
Familial PDAC	Unknown	Varies with # FDRs with PDAC[50]	Not applicable	Start at age 50 y or 10 y younger than the earliest diagnosis in the family

Abbreviations: SDR, second-degree relative.
[a] Adapted from the CAPS consortium[51] and NCCN guidelines.[10]

an absolute rate of 118.6 cases of PDAC per 100,000 person-years, corresponding with a cumulative risk of 36% by age 64.[20]

Familial Atypical Mole and Multiple Melanoma Syndrome

Familial atypical mole and multiple melanoma (FAMMM) syndrome is an autosomal-dominant syndrome diagnosed in individuals with a personal history of more than 50 atypical nevi and a family history of melanoma. FAMMM is most commonly caused by pathogenic alterations in the cell cycle gene *CDKN2A*, a gene which encodes for p16 and p14ARF.

The association of FAMMM with PDAC was first reported in 1991, although families with coexisting melanoma and PDAC were reported 20 years earlier.[21] An analysis of the Dutch FAMMM registry identified a specific 19 base-pair deletion in exon 2 of *CDKN2A* ("p16-Leiden") that conferred a risk of PDAC of 17% by age 75.[22] The age specific risk was less than 1% for carriers at age 40 years and 4% at age 50 years. Smoking further modifies these risks.[23]

In a large PDAC cohort, the prevalence of *CDKN2A* mutations was 0.6%, including 3.3% among those with an FDR affected with PDAC and 5.3% with FDR with melanoma.[24] Consistent with this study, *CDKN2A* mutations have been identified in other unselected PDAC cohorts at a frequency of 0.3% to 0.7%.[5,8,9]

BRCA-Associated Cancer

BRCA-associated cancers include breast, ovarian, pancreatic and prostate cancer. BRCA-associated cancer is often referred to as hereditary breast and ovarian cancer, an autosomal-dominant syndrome caused by pathogenic alterations in *BRCA1* and *BRCA2*. *BRCA1* and *BRCA2* mutations are present in about 1 out of every 40 Ashkenazi Jews[25] and in about 1 out of every 300 to 465 women in the general population.[26] Both *BRCA1* and *BRCA2* are tumor suppressor genes involved in homologous recombination, a form of DNA repair.

The association of *BRCA* alterations with PDAC was noted as early as 1996[27] with larger cohort studies subsequently identifying an increased risk for PDAC among both *BRCA1* (2.3 fold)[28] and *BRCA2* (3.5–6 fold) mutation carriers.[29,30] *BRCA2* alterations are one of the most common cancer predisposition genes identified on germline genetic testing with rates of 1.3% to 3.6%[5,6,8,9,31] among unselected patients with PDAC, and approximately double this rate[32,33] among cohorts with FPC and/or Ashkenazi Jewish ancestry. The frequency of *BRCA1* mutation carriers identified in unselected PDAC cohorts is 0.3% to 1.3%.[5,8,9,31]

Among *BRCA*-associated cancers that have deficient homologous recombination, treatment with PARP inhibitors can selectively induce tumor cell death.[11] PARP inhibitors are currently approved by the US Food and Drug Administration for specific settings for *BRCA*-associated ovarian (first approved in 2014), breast (2018), pancreatic (2019), and prostate (2020) cancers.

Lynch Syndrome

The Lynch syndrome is an autosomal-dominant cancer predisposition syndrome caused by pathogenic alterations in mismatch repair genes (*MLH1*, *MSH2*, *MSH6*, and *PMS2*) and *EPCAM* with an estimated population prevalence of 1 in 279.[34] Lynch carriers are at increased lifetime risk for a wide spectrum of cancers, most commonly colorectal and endometrial cancers, but also ovarian, urinary tract, gastric, small bowel, brain, sebaceous neoplasms, and PDACs.[35]

In a study including 147 Lynch syndrome (*MLH1, MSH2,* and *MSH6*) mutation carriers, 21% had at least 1 family member with PDAC.[36] The same study found a 1.3% cumulative risk for developing PDAC by age 50%, and 3.7% risk by age 70.

Lynch syndrome-associated cancers characteristically possess microsatellite instability (changes in lengths of repetitive DNA sequences) as a result of defective mismatch repair. Microsatellite instability–high and mismatch repair deficient tumors can be identified by evaluating tumor tissue with immunohistochemistry for the presence or absence of the MLH1, MSH2, MSH6, and PMS2 proteins, microsatellite instability testing, or next-generation DNA sequencing.[37–39] Patients with PDACs that are microsatellite instability–high or mismatch repair deficient are candidates for treatment with immune checkpoint inhibitors.[12]

ATM

ATM encodes for a protein important in DNA strand break repair. Homozygous *ATM* alterations lead to the syndrome of ataxia–telangiectasia, an autosomal-recessive condition characterized by ataxia, increased sensitivity to radiation, and a more than 100-fold increased risk of hematologic malignancies and other cancers.[40] Germline *ATM* mutations are significantly more common in patients with FPC compared with controls.[41] Heterozygote *ATM* carriers are at increased risk for developing cancer, including a moderate increased risk of breast and PDAC, with possible risks for colon, prostate, and ovarian cancers.[41,42] One large case-control study found a 5.7-fold increased odds of having *ATM* mutations in sporadic PDAC cases compared with controls.[8] In cohorts of unselected patients with PDAC, *ATM* variants have been identified in 1.2% to 3.3%.[5,6,8,9]

PALB2

The partner and localizer of BRCA2 (*PALB2*) gene encodes a protein that interacts with and stabilizes the BRCA2 protein, with an overlap in cancer predisposition between *BRCA2* and *PALB2* pathogenic variants. In an international study of 524 families with *PALB2* alterations, the risk to age 80 years for female breast cancer was 53%, 5% for ovarian (relative risk, 2.91), 2% to 3% for pancreatic (relative risk, 2.37), and 1% for male breast cancer (relative risk, 7.34).[43] *PALB2* mutations have been identified in 3% to 4% of familial[44,45] and 0.2 to 0.4% of unselected PDAC cohorts.[5,6,8,9]

Li–Fraumeni Syndrome

Li–Fraumeni syndrome is an autosomal-dominant, highly penetrant syndrome caused by germline mutations in the *TP53* gene, a tumor suppressor gene that regulates many processes involved in cell cycle and DNA repair. The estimated prevalence is about 1 in every 3500 to 5500 individuals,[46] and an analysis of 286 patients with Li–Fraumeni syndrome in the National Cancer Institute (NCI) Li–Fraumeni syndrome study reported a cancer incidence of almost 100% for both sexes by age 70, but only 5 PDACs.[47] In cohorts of unselected patients with PDAC, *TP53* mutations have been identified in 0.12% to 0.50%.[5–7,48]

Familial pancreatic ductal adenocarcinoma

FPC kindreds are defined as those families with at least 2 FDRs with PDAC, without a known predisposing genetic mutation. In fact, in 1 study including 185 patients with FPC, less than 15% were found to have informative germline testing.[49] Even in the absence of an identifiable pathogenic mutation, FPC kindred patients are at increased risk for PDAC. An analysis of the prospective National Familial Pancreas Tumor Registry compared the number of PDACs observed to the expected number using NCI Surveillance Epidemiology and End Results (SEER) incidence rates and found that members of FPC kindreds with 1 FDR had 4.6-fold (95% confidence interval, 0.5–16.4) increased risk, 2 FDRs had a 6.4-fold (95% confidence interval, 1.8–16.4) increased risk, and those with 3 or more FDRs had a 32-fold (95% confidence interval, 10.2–74.7) increased risk compared with SEER incidence rates.[50]

GOALS OF PANCREATIC SURVEILLANCE

The International Cancer of the Pancreas Screening (CAPS) Consortium proposed the primary objectives for PDAC surveillance as the detection and treatment of stage I PDAC and PDAC precursor lesions with high-grade dysplasia, including pancreatic intraepithelial neoplasia and intraductal papillary mucinous neoplasms.[51] Surveillance is associated with downstaging of diagnosed PDACs, especially among those who maintain an annual surveillance schedule.[52,53] Recent analysis of NCI SEER data found survival of stage I PDAC has been improving, with an 80% survival at 5 years among patients who undergo pancreatic resection, highlighting the potential of early detection strategies.[54]

WHOM TO SCREEN AND WHEN

The US Preventative Task Force recommends against screening for PDAC in asymptomatic adults in the general population, given no evidence for a decrease in mortality and the potential for greater harm than benefit.[3] Importantly, this recommendation does not apply to those individuals at high risk owing to genetics and/or family history. Multiple professional society guidelines now recommend surveillance[10,51,55,56] specifically for individuals with (1) PJS, FAMMM, or HP, (2) inherited pathogenic alterations in *ATM, BRCA1, BRCA2, MLH1, MSH2, MSH6, PALB2*, or *TP53* and a family history of PDAC in at least 1 FDR[51] or second-degree relative (SDR),[10] and (3) FPC with at least 1 FDR and 1 SDR with PDAC. The presence of a single FDR or SDR with PDAC (in the absence of a known genetic mutation or inherited PDAC risk syndrome) is not sufficient to recommend surveillance.

When PDAC screening is indicated, the optimal age to begin screening is not well-established. Consensus guidelines from the CAPS Consortium[51] and National Comprehensive Cancer Network[10] recommend a gene/syndrome-specific approach. Carriers of high-risk genes or genetic syndromes (owing to mutations in *ATM, BRCA1, BRCA2, MLH1, MSH2, MSH6, PALB2*, or *TP53*) with at least 1 FDR[51] or SDR[10] with PDAC may begin screening at age 50 years or 10 years younger than the earliest PDAC in the family (whichever is earliest). Screening should begin at a younger age for patients with PJS (age 30–35 years) and HP (age 40 years or 20 years after onset of pancreatitis) and *CDKN2A* mutation carriers (age 40 years or within 10 years of the earliest PDAC in the family). It is also not well-established when or at what age screening should be discontinued, and this decision requires consideration of a patient's comorbidities and life expectancy, perceived cancer risk, and personal preferences. In general, it is important that providers have an informed discussion with patients before starting a surveillance program.

METHODS OF SCREENING
Visualization of the Pancreas

Professional society guidelines recommend a combination of EUS examination and MRI/MR cholangiopancreatography to evaluate the pancreas in appropriate high-risk individuals.[10,51,57] In a multicenter blinded study evaluating the diagnostic yield of EUS examination and MRI, EUS examination was found to be more sensitive for the detection of small, solid lesions and chronic pancreatic type parenchymal changes, whereas MRI was more sensitive for detection of small, cystic lesions, suggesting an additive rather than duplicative effect of the 2 imaging techniques.[58] In another study where patients underwent computed tomography (CT) scanning, MRI, and EUS examination, CT imaging often missed subcentimeter pancreatic cysts detected by MRI and EUS examination.[59] Given the complementary information provided by MRI and EUS examination, neither of which exposes patients to radiation, these modalities are preferentially used for routine high-risk pancreatic screening.

Among patients without concerning features on baseline imaging, alternating EUS and MRI screening may be performed annually (**Fig. 1**).[51] The CAPS guidelines recommend that, for concerning abnormalities (cysts with worrisome features, solid lesions, main pancreatic duct stricture and/or dilation of $\geq$6 mm without a mass), EUS examination with fine needle aspiration and/or CT imaging be obtained.[51] Surveillance intervals should be shortened when worrisome features are present without clear evidence of cancer (3–6 months rather than every 12 months).[51] Importantly, physician discretion and clinical concern based on patient characteristics and family history should be incorporated into the surveillance paradigm for all high-risk patients.

Biomarkers

In middle-aged and older adults, new-onset diabetes (NOD) can be a harbinger of PDAC. In a population based study of 2122 individuals with diabetes diagnosed at 50 years of age or older, 0.85% were diagnosed with PDAC within 3 years of diabetes diagnosis.[60] Similarly, in a prospective cohort study of 112,818 individuals from the Nurses' Health Study and Health Professionals Follow-Up Study, NOD was associated with an increased risk of PDAC, and this risk was higher still in patients with NOD accompanied by unintentional weight loss and older age.[61] Although NOD and monitoring of fasting blood sugar or hemoglobin A1c have not been evaluated extensively in populations with inherited PDAC syndromes, the CAPS consortium guidelines recommend serial measurement of fasting glucose and/or hemoglobin A1c, with rising blood glucose suggestive of the need for closer surveillance.[51]

Carbohydrate antigen 19-9 (CA19-9) is a serum biomarker that has been associated with PDAC disease stage, overall survival time and response to treatment. The use of CA19-9 for general population screening is not recommended. However, in a multi-institutional analysis, elevation of CA19-9 had a sensitivity of 64% at 99% specificity for newly diagnosed resectable PDAC compared with healthy controls.[62] Elevated CA19-9 levels were also detected in the year before a PDAC diagnosis, with a sensitivity of 60% at 99% specificity within the 6 months before a diagnosis.[62] Similar results were found in a large study comparing subjects undergoing pancreatic surveillance with those with early-stage PDAC.[63] The CAPS consortium recommends considering measurement of CA19-9 at the time of enhanced clinical concern for PDAC, such as with worrisome findings on imaging.[51]

OUTCOMES FROM SURVEILLANCE
Results from Imaging Surveillance

Small cysts are common (>40%) among patients with inherited PDAC syndrome undergoing surveillance,[59] although the vast majority are not worrisome or at significant risk of neoplastic transformation. The pattern of cysts or lesions may differ in size or progression risk depending on the underlying predisposition prompting screening,[64] and germline mutation carriers are at higher risk for high-grade dysplasia or cancer compared with patients with FPC without known mutation.[65]

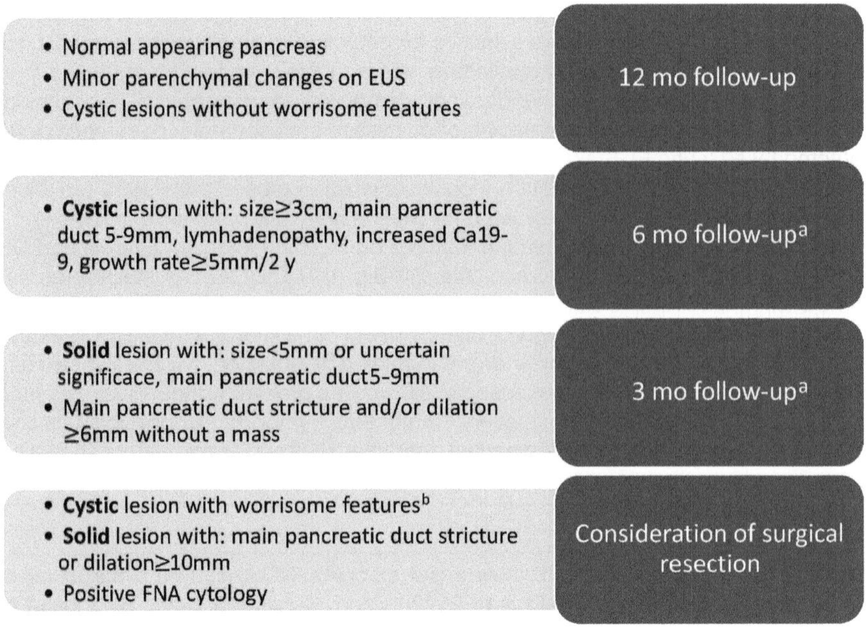

• Normal appearing pancreas • Minor parenchymal changes on EUS • Cystic lesions without worrisome features	12 mo follow-up
• **Cystic** lesion with: size≥3cm, main pancreatic duct 5-9mm, lymhadenopathy, increased Ca19-9, growth rate≥5mm/2 y	6 mo follow-up[a]
• **Solid** lesion with: size<5mm or uncertain significace, main pancreatic duct5-9mm • Main pancreatic duct stricture and/or dilation ≥6mm without a mass	3 mo follow-up[a]
• **Cystic** lesion with worrisome features[b] • **Solid** lesion with: main pancreatic duct stricture or dilation≥10mm • Positive FNA cytology	Consideration of surgical resection

Fig. 1. Approach to surveillance intervals for high-risk pancreatic cancer screening (per CAPS Consortium guidelines). FNA, fine needle aspiration. [a]For concerning features (including findings listed in the 6-month follow-up and 3-month follow-up boxes), fine needle aspiration and/or CT imaging should be considered to better characterize the lesion and assess risk for malignancy. In addition to MRI and EUS findings, patient-specific risk factors (including clinical factors and family history) may also be incorporated into risk assessment and lead to earlier tissue sampling or more frequent follow-up per provider discretion. [b]Worrisome features of cystic lesions include a mural nodule, enhanced solid component, thickened or enhanced cyst walls, abrupt main pancreatic duct caliber change or size 10 mm or greater, or patient symptoms (pancreatitis, jaundice, pain).

Imaging and Clinical Features Associated with Progression

Just as there are certain worrisome features seen on pancreas imaging among the general population that require monitoring or other intervention,[66] certain imaging findings in inherited PDAC syndrome patients may necessitate shorter follow-up or intervention owing to risk of neoplastic progression (see **Fig. 1**). In a CAPS analysis of 354 high-risk patients, 24 (7%) had progression (10 high-grade dysplasia, 14 pancreatic adenocarcinoma) over 16 years of evaluation.[53] This finding corresponds with a 1.6% per year progression rate, with 93% of patients having a worrisome finding before being diagnosed with high-grade dysplasia or adenocarcinoma.[53]

Surgical Outcomes and Survival

The decision to pursue surgical intervention requires multidisciplinary review and evaluation of patient specific factors. Because surgery remains the only treatment with the potential to cure PDAC, the goal of surveillance is to detect high-risk precursors or stage I invasive cancer that can be removed surgically. In a series of 10 PDACs detected during surveillance of 354 high-risk patients, 9 had an R0 resection and 90% were alive at 1 year with 60% alive at 5 years.[67] Another analysis of 71 patients who underwent pancreatic resection during surveillance found no difference in survival between those with low-risk and high-risk precursors, although survival was poorer in those diagnosed with pancreatic adenocarcinoma.[68] A meta-analysis of high-risk cohort studies found 253 to 281 high-risk patients would need to be screened to prevent 1 death from PDAC,[69] although further studies are needed to confirm these results.

FUTURE INVESTIGATIONS
New Pancreatic Ductal Adenocarcinoma Susceptibility Genes

Germline genetic testing is now recommended for all patients diagnosed with PDAC,[10] and the number of genes evaluated will continue to expand as researchers study PDAC-prone families. For example, whole-genome sequencing of 1 such family led to the identification of a germline truncating mutation in the *RABL3* gene, which alters RAS pathway regulation.[70] Additionally, genome wide association studies have identified common genetic variants that predispose to PDAC with much lower penetrance, but may ultimately allow for clinically meaningful risk stratification using calculated genetic risk scores.[71–73]

New Methods for Earlier Pancreatic Ductal Adenocarcinoma Detection

The development of new circulating biomarkers for the early detection of PDAC remains an active area of investigation. A number of tests are in development that measure circulating tumor DNA, proteins, metabolites, and other types of markers in the blood.[74,75] Other approaches are evaluating pancreatic juice, including with next-generation DNA sequencing to detect mutations associated with high-grade dysplasia or invasive cancer.[76] Molecular analysis of pancreatic cyst fluid is also being evaluated for its utility to distinguishing cysts that require resection, surveillance, or neither.[77]

SUMMARY

For the subset of individuals at increased risk of PDAC owing to an inherited PDAC syndrome, PDAC surveillance holds promise as a way to improve survival by detecting and intervening on noninvasive dysplastic precursors or early cancers. Further studies are required to define more clearly the appropriate populations for screening and quantify the benefits and risks of screening programs.

CLINICS CARE POINTS

- PDAC has poor overall survival and is often diagnosed at an advanced stage.
- Individuals with inherited PDAC syndromes may benefit from PDAC surveillance.
- For most patients, surveillance involves annual pancreatic imaging using EUS examination and MRI/MR cholangiopancreatography, which provide complementary views of the pancreas and are the current standard of care for PDAC screening.
- The goal of PDAC surveillance is to detect and intervene early upon high-risk noninvasive precursors or early-stage cancers. Although surveillance has not been definitively shown to improve survival, it is associated with a downstaging of detected PDACs, and efforts are ongoing to refine surveillance approaches and understand their potential benefits.

FUNDING SUPPORT

BMW is supported by the Hale Family Center for Pancreatic Cancer Research, Lustgarten Foundation Dedicated Laboratory program, NIH grant U01 CA210171, NIH grant P50 CA127003, Stand Up to Cancer, Pancreatic Cancer Action Network, Noble Effort Fund, Wexler Family Fund, and Promises for Purple. Michael Goggins is supported by the National Cancer Institute (U01210170, CA62924 and R01CA176828 and by a Stand Up To Cancer-Lustgarten Foundation Pancreatic Cancer Interception Translational Cancer Research Grant (Grant Number: SU2C-AACR-DT25-17). Stand Up To Cancer is a program of the Entertainment Industry Foundation. SU2C research grants are administered by the American Association for Cancer Research, the scientific partner of SU2C.

DISCLOSURES

BMW declares grant funding from Celgene and Eli Lilly, and consulting for BioLineRx, Celgene, and GRAIL.

REFERENCES

1. Siegel RL, Miller KD, Jemal A. Cancer statistics, 2020. CA Cancer J Clin 2020; 70(1):7–30.
2. National Cancer Institute. Cancer stat facts: pancreatic cancer. Available at: https://seer.cancer.gov/statfacts/html/pancreas.html. Accessed December 5, 2020.
3. U.S Preventive Services Task Force, Owens DK, Davidson KW, Krist AH, et al. Screening for pancreatic cancer: US Preventive Services Task Force reaffirmation recommendation statement. JAMA 2019;322(5):438–44.
4. Roberts NJ, Norris AL, Petersen GM, et al. Whole genome sequencing defines the genetic heterogeneity of familial pancreatic cancer. Cancer Discov 2016; 6(2):166–75.
5. Yurgelun MB, Chittenden AB, Morales-Oyarvide V, et al. Germline cancer susceptibility gene variants, somatic second hits, and survival outcomes in patients with resected pancreatic cancer. Genet Med 2019;21(1):213–23.
6. Shindo K, Yu J, Suenaga M, et al. Deleterious germline mutations in patients with apparently sporadic pancreatic adenocarcinoma. J Clin Oncol 2017;35(30): 3382–90.
7. Lowery MA, Wong W, Jordan EJ, et al. Prospective evaluation of germline alterations in patients with exocrine pancreatic neoplasms. J Natl Cancer Inst 2018; 110(10):1067–74.
8. Hu C, Hart SN, Polley EC, et al. Association between inherited germline mutations in cancer predisposition genes and risk of pancreatic cancer. JAMA 2018; 319(23):2401–9.
9. Brand R, Borazanci E, Speare V, et al. Prospective study of germline genetic testing in incident cases of pancreatic adenocarcinoma. Cancer 2018;124(17): 3520–7.
10. NCCN Guidelines Version 2. Genetic/family high-risk assessment: breast, ovarian, and pancreatic. 2021. Available at: https://www.nccn.org/professionals/physician_gls/pdf/genetics_bop.pdf. Accessed December 20, 2020.
11. Golan T, Hammel P, Reni M, et al. Maintenance olaparib for germline BRCA-mutated metastatic pancreatic cancer. N Engl J Med 2019;381(4):317–27.

12. Marabelle A, Le DT, Ascierto PA, et al. Efficacy of pembrolizumab in patients with noncolorectal high microsatellite instability/mismatch repair-deficient cancer: results from the phase II KEYNOTE-158 study. J Clin Oncol 2020;38(1):1–10.

13. Lowenfels AB, Maisonneuve P, DiMagno EP, et al. Hereditary pancreatitis and the risk of pancreatic cancer. International Hereditary Pancreatitis Study Group. J Natl Cancer Inst 1997;89(6):442–6.

14. Shelton CA, Umapathy C, Stello K, et al. Hereditary pancreatitis in the United States: survival and rates of pancreatic cancer. Am J Gastroenterol 2018; 113(9):1376.

15. Lowenfels AB, Maisonneuve P, Whitcomb DC, et al. Cigarette smoking as a risk factor for pancreatic cancer in patients with hereditary pancreatitis. JAMA 2001;286(2):169–70.

16. Tamura K, Yu J, Hata T, et al. Mutations in the pancreatic secretory enzymes CPA1 and CPB1 are associated with pancreatic cancer. Proc Natl Acad Sci U S A 2018;115(18):4767–72.

17. Rebours V, Boutron-Ruault MC, Schnee M, et al. The natural history of hereditary pancreatitis: a national series. Gut 2009;58(1):97–103.

18. van Lier MG, Wagner A, Mathus-Vliegen EM, et al. High cancer risk in Peutz-Jeghers syndrome: a systematic review and surveillance recommendations. Am J Gastroenterol 2010;105(6):1258–64, author reply 1265.

19. Hearle N, Schumacher V, Menko FH, et al. Frequency and spectrum of cancers in the Peutz-Jeghers syndrome. Clin Cancer Res 2006;12(10):3209–15.

20. Giardiello FM, Brensinger JD, Tersmette AC, et al. Very high risk of cancer in familial Peutz-Jeghers syndrome. Gastroenterology 2000;119(6):1447–53.

21. Lynch HT, Shaw TG. Familial atypical multiple mole melanoma (FAMMM) syndrome: history, genetics, and heterogeneity. Fam Cancer 2016;15(3):487–91.

22. Vasen HF, Gruis NA, Frants RR, et al. Risk of developing pancreatic cancer in families with familial atypical multiple mole melanoma associated with a specific 19 deletion of p16 (p16-Leiden). Int J Cancer 2000;87(6):809–11.

23. Potjer TP, Kranenburg HE, Bergman W, et al. Prospective risk of cancer and the influence of tobacco use in carriers of the p16-Leiden germline variant. Eur J Hum Genet 2015;23(5):711–4.

24. McWilliams RR, Wieben ED, Rabe KG, et al. Prevalence of CDKN2A mutations in pancreatic cancer patients: implications for genetic counseling. Eur J Hum Genet 2011;19(4):472–8.

25. Roa BB, Boyd AA, Volcik K, et al. Ashkenazi Jewish population frequencies for common mutations in BRCA1 and BRCA2. Nat Genet 1996;14(2):185–7.

26. McClain MR, Palomaki GE, Nathanson KL, et al. Adjusting the estimated proportion of breast cancer cases associated with BRCA1 and BRCA2 mutations: public health implications. Genet Med 2005;7(1):28–33.

27. Goggins M, Schutte M, Lu J, et al. Germline BRCA2 gene mutations in patients with apparently sporadic pancreatic carcinomas. Cancer Res 1996;56(23): 5360–4.

28. Thompson D, Easton DF, Breast Cancer Linkage C. Cancer incidence in BRCA1 mutation carriers. J Natl Cancer Inst 2002;94(18):1358–65.

29. Breast Cancer Linkage C. Cancer risks in BRCA2 mutation carriers. J Natl Cancer Inst 1999;91(15):1310–6.

30. van Asperen CJ, Brohet RM, Meijers-Heijboer EJ, et al. Cancer risks in BRCA2 families: estimates for sites other than breast and ovary. J Med Genet 2005; 42(9):711–9.

31. Holter S, Borgida A, Dodd A, et al. Germline BRCA mutations in a large clinic-based cohort of patients with pancreatic adenocarcinoma. J Clin Oncol 2015; 33(28):3124–9.

32. Ferrone CR, Levine DA, Tang LH, et al. BRCA germline mutations in Jewish patients with pancreatic adenocarcinoma. J Clin Oncol 2009;27(3):433–8.

33. Zhen DB, Rabe KG, Gallinger S, et al. BRCA1, BRCA2, PALB2, and CDKN2A mutations in familial pancreatic cancer: a PACGENE study. Genet Med 2015;17(7): 569–77.

34. Win AK, Jenkins MA, Dowty JG, et al. Prevalence and penetrance of major genes and polygenes for colorectal cancer. Cancer Epidemiol Biomarkers Prev 2017; 26(3):404–12.

35. Dominguez-Valentin M, Sampson JR, Seppala TT, et al. Cancer risks by gene, age, and gender in 6350 carriers of pathogenic mismatch repair variants: findings from the Prospective Lynch Syndrome Database. Genet Med 2020;22(1): 15–25.

36. Kastrinos F, Mukherjee B, Tayob N, et al. Risk of pancreatic cancer in families with Lynch syndrome. JAMA 2009;302(16):1790–5.

37. Aguirre AJ, Nowak JA, Camarda ND, et al. Real-time genomic characterization of advanced pancreatic cancer to enable precision medicine. Cancer Discov 2018; 8(9):1096–111.

38. Hu ZI, Shia J, Stadler ZK, et al. Evaluating mismatch repair deficiency in pancreatic adenocarcinoma: challenges and recommendations. Clin Cancer Res 2018; 24(6):1326–36.

39. Grant RC, Denroche R, Jang GH, et al. Clinical and genomic characterisation of mismatch repair deficient pancreatic adenocarcinoma. Gut 2020;15: 2020-320730.

40. Morrell D, Cromartie E, Swift M. Mortality and cancer incidence in 263 patients with ataxia-telangiectasia. J Natl Cancer Inst 1986;77(1):89–92.

41. Roberts NJ, Jiao Y, Yu J, et al. ATM mutations in patients with hereditary pancreatic cancer. Cancer Discov 2012;2(1):41–6.

42. van Os NJ, Roeleveld N, Weemaes CM, et al. Health risks for ataxia-telangiectasia mutated heterozygotes: a systematic review, meta-analysis and evidence-based guideline. Clin Genet 2016;90(2):105–17.

43. Yang X, Leslie G, Doroszuk A, et al. Cancer risks associated with germline palb2 pathogenic variants: an international study of 524 families. J Clin Oncol 2020; 38(7):674–85.

44. Jones S, Hruban RH, Kamiyama M, et al. Exomic sequencing identifies PALB2 as a pancreatic cancer susceptibility gene. Science 2009;324(5924):217.

45. Slater EP, Langer P, Niemczyk E, et al. PALB2 mutations in European familial pancreatic cancer families. Clin Genet 2010;78(5):490–4.

46. de Andrade KC, Frone MN, Wegman-Ostrosky T, et al. Variable population prevalence estimates of germline TP53 variants: a gnomAD-based analysis. Hum Mutat 2019;40(1):97–105.

47. Mai PL, Best AF, Peters JA, et al. Risks of first and subsequent cancers among TP53 mutation carriers in the National Cancer Institute Li-Fraumeni syndrome cohort. Cancer 2016;122(23):3673–81.

48. Grant RC, Selander I, Connor AA, et al. Prevalence of germline mutations in cancer predisposition genes in patients with pancreatic cancer. Gastroenterology 2015;148(3):556–64.

49. Chaffee KG, Oberg AL, McWilliams RR, et al. Prevalence of germ-line mutations in cancer genes among pancreatic cancer patients with a positive family history. Genet Med 2018;20(1):119–27.
50. Klein AP, Brune KA, Petersen GM, et al. Prospective risk of pancreatic cancer in familial pancreatic cancer kindreds. Cancer Res 2004;64(7):2634–8.
51. Goggins M, Overbeek KA, Brand R, et al. Management of patients with increased risk for familial pancreatic cancer: updated recommendations from the International Cancer of the Pancreas Screening (CAPS) Consortium. Gut 2020; 69(1):7–17.
52. Vasen H, Ibrahim I, Ponce CG, et al. Benefit of surveillance for pancreatic cancer in high-risk individuals: outcome of long-term prospective follow-up studies from three European expert centers. J Clin Oncol 2016;34(17):2010–9.
53. Canto MI, Almario JA, Schulick RD, et al. Risk of neoplastic progression in individuals at high risk for pancreatic cancer undergoing long-term surveillance. Gastroenterology 2018;155(3):740–51.e2.
54. Blackford AL, Canto MI, Klein AP, et al. Recent trends in the incidence and survival of stage 1A pancreatic cancer: a surveillance, epidemiology, and end results analysis. J Natl Cancer Inst 2020;112(5709818):1162–9.
55. Stoffel EM, McKernin SE, Brand R, et al. Evaluating susceptibility to pancreatic cancer: ASCO provisional clinical opinion. J Clin Oncol 2019;37(2):153–64.
56. Stjepanovic N, Moreira L, Carneiro F, et al. Hereditary gastrointestinal cancers: ESMO clinical practice guidelines for diagnosis, treatment and follow-up. Ann Oncol 2019;30(10):1558–71.
57. Aslanian HR, Lee JH, Canto MI. AGA clinical practice update on pancreas cancer screening in high-risk individuals: expert review. Gastroenterology 2020; 159(1):358–62.
58. Harinck F, Konings IC, Kluijt I, et al. A multicentre comparative prospective blinded analysis of EUS and MRI for screening of pancreatic cancer in high-risk individuals. Gut 2016;65(9):1505–13.
59. Canto MI, Hruban RH, Fishman EK, et al. Frequent detection of pancreatic lesions in asymptomatic high-risk individuals. Gastroenterology 2012;142(4):796–804 [quiz e714-95].
60. Chari ST, Leibson CL, Rabe KG, et al. Probability of pancreatic cancer following diabetes: a population-based study. Gastroenterology 2005;129(2):504–11.
61. Yuan C, Babic A, Khalaf N, et al. Diabetes, weight change, and pancreatic cancer risk. JAMA Oncol 2020;6(10):e202948.
62. Fahrmann JF, Schmidt CM, Mao X, et al. Lead-Time Trajectory of CA19-9 as an Anchor Marker for Pancreatic Cancer Early Detection. Gastroenterology 2021; 160. https://doi.org/10.1053/j.gastro.2020.11.052. 1373-1383.e6.
63. Abe T, Koi C, Kohi S, et al. That Affect Levels of Circulating Tumor Markers Increase Identification of Patients With Pancreatic Cancer. Clin Gastroenterol Hepatol 2020. https://doi.org/10.1016/j.cgh.2019.10.036. 1161-1169.e5.
64. Konings IC, Harinck F, Poley JW, et al. Prevalence and progression of pancreatic cystic precursor lesions differ between groups at high risk of developing pancreatic cancer. Pancreas 2017;46(1):28–34.
65. Abe T, Blackford AL, Tamura K, et al. Deleterious germline mutations are a risk factor for neoplastic progression among high-risk individuals undergoing pancreatic surveillance. J Clin Oncol 2019;37(13):1070–80.
66. Tanaka M, Fernandez-Del Castillo C, Kamisawa T, et al. Revisions of international consensus Fukuoka guidelines for the management of IPMN of the pancreas. Pancreatology 2017;17(5):738–53.

67. Canto MI, Kerdsirichairat T, Yeo CJ, et al. Surgical outcomes after pancreatic resection of screening-detected lesions in individuals at high risk for developing pancreatic cancer. J Gastrointest Surg 2020;24(5):1101–10.

68. Konings I, Canto MI, Almario JA, et al. Surveillance for pancreatic cancer in high-risk individuals. BJS Open 2019;3(5):656–65.

69. Corral JE, Mareth KF, Riegert-Johnson DL, et al. Diagnostic yield from screening asymptomatic individuals at high risk for pancreatic cancer: a meta-analysis of cohort studies. Clin Gastroenterol Hepatol 2019;17(1):41–53.

70. Nissim S, Leshchiner I, Mancias JD, et al. Mutations in RABL3 alter KRAS prenylation and are associated with hereditary pancreatic cancer. Nat Genet 2019; 51(9):1308–14.

71. Klein AP, Wolpin BM, Risch HA, et al. Genome-wide meta-analysis identifies five new susceptibility loci for pancreatic cancer. Nat Commun 2018;9(1):556.

72. Wolpin BM, Rizzato C, Kraft P, et al. Genome-wide association study identifies multiple susceptibility loci for pancreatic cancer. Nat Genet 2014;46(9): 994–1000.

73. Kim J, Yuan C, Babic A, et al. Genetic and circulating biomarker data improve risk prediction for pancreatic cancer in the general population. Cancer Epidemiol Biomarkers Prev 2020;29(5):999–1008.

74. Cohen JD, Li L, Wang Y, et al. Detection and localization of surgically resectable cancers with a multi-analyte blood test. Science 2018;359(6378):926–30.

75. Liu MC, Oxnard GR, Klein EA, et al. Sensitive and specific multi-cancer detection and localization using methylation signatures in cell-free DNA. Ann Oncol 2020; 31(6):745–59.

76. Suenaga M, Yu J, Shindo K, et al. Pancreatic juice mutation concentrations can help predict the grade of dysplasia in patients undergoing pancreatic surveillance. Clin Cancer Res 2018;24(12):2963–74.

77. Springer S, Masica DL, Dal Molin M, et al. A multimodality test to guide the management of patients with a pancreatic cyst. Sci Transl Med 2019;11(501): eaav4772.

78. Brose MS, Rebbeck TR, Calzone KA, et al. Cancer risk estimates for BRCA1 mutation carriers identified in a risk evaluation program. J Natl Cancer Inst 2002; 94(18):1365–72.

UNITED STATES POSTAL SERVICE ® Statement of Ownership, Management, and Circulation
(All Periodicals Publications Except Requester Publications)

1. Publication Title	2. Publication Number	3. Filing Date
SURGICAL ONCOLOGY CLINICS OF NORTH AMERICA	012 – 565	9/18/2021

4. Issue Frequency	5. Number of Issues Published Annually	6. Annual Subscription Price
JAN, APR, JUL, OCT	4	$315.00

7. Complete Mailing Address of Known Office of Publication (Not printer) (Street, city, county, state, and ZIP+4®)
ELSEVIER INC.
230 Park Avenue, Suite 800
New York, NY 10169

Contact Person
Malathi Samayan

Telephone (include area code)
91-44-4299-4507

8. Complete Mailing Address of Headquarters or General Business Office of Publisher (Not printer)
ELSEVIER INC.
230 Park Avenue, Suite 800
New York, NY 10169

9. Full Names and Complete Mailing Addresses of Publisher, Editor, and Managing Editor (Do not leave blank)

Publisher (Name and complete mailing address)
DOLORES MELONI, ELSEVIER INC.
1600 JOHN F KENNEDY BLVD. SUITE 1800
PHILADELPHIA, PA 19103-2899

Editor (Name and complete mailing address)
JOHN VASSALLO, ELSEVIER INC.
1600 JOHN F KENNEDY BLVD. SUITE 1800
PHILADELPHIA, PA 19103-2899

Managing Editor (Name and complete mailing address)
PATRICK MANLEY, ELSEVIER INC.
1600 JOHN F KENNEDY BLVD. SUITE 1800
PHILADELPHIA, PA 19103-2899

10. Owner (Do not leave blank. If the publication is owned by a corporation, give the name and address of the corporation immediately followed by the names and addresses of all stockholders owning or holding 1 percent or more of the total amount of stock. If not owned by a corporation, give the names and addresses of the individual owners. If owned by a partnership or other unincorporated firm, give its name and address as well as those of each individual owner. If the publication is published by a nonprofit organization, give its name and address.)

Full Name	Complete Mailing Address
WHOLLY OWNED SUBSIDIARY OF REED/ELSEVIER, US HOLDINGS	1600 JOHN F KENNEDY BLVD. SUITE 1800 PHILADELPHIA, PA 19103-2899

11. Known Bondholders, Mortgagees, and Other Security Holders Owning or Holding 1 Percent or More of Total Amount of Bonds, Mortgages, or Other Securities. If none, check box ▶ ☐ None

Full Name	Complete Mailing Address
N/A	

12. Tax Status (For completion by nonprofit organizations authorized to mail at nonprofit rates) (Check one)
The purpose, function, and nonprofit status of this organization and the exempt status for federal income tax purposes:
☒ Has Not Changed During Preceding 12 Months
☐ Has Changed During Preceding 12 Months (Publisher must submit explanation of change with this statement)

PS Form 3526, July 2014 [Page 1 of 4 (see instructions page 4)] PSN 7530-01-000-9931 PRIVACY NOTICE: See our privacy policy on www.usps.com.

---

13. Publication Title	14. Issue Date for Circulation Data Below
SURGICAL ONCOLOGY CLINICS OF NORTH AMERICA	JULY 2021

15. Extent and Nature of Circulation			Average No. Copies Each Issue During Preceding 12 Months	No. Copies of Single Issue Published Nearest to Filing Date
a. Total Number of Copies (Net press run)			102	98
b. Paid Circulation (By Mail and Outside the Mail)	(1)	Mailed Outside-County Paid Subscriptions Stated on PS Form 3541 (include paid distribution above nominal rate, advertiser's proof copies, and exchange copies)	41	36
	(2)	Mailed In-County Paid Subscriptions Stated on PS Form 3541 (include paid distribution above nominal rate, advertiser's proof copies, and exchange copies)	0	0
	(3)	Paid Distribution Outside the Mails Including Sales Through Dealers and Carriers, Street Vendors, Counter Sales, and Other Paid Distribution Outside USPS®	32	34
	(4)	Paid Distribution by Other Classes of Mail Through the USPS (e.g., First-Class Mail®)	0	0
c. Total Paid Distribution (Sum of 15b (1), (2), (3), and (4))			73	70
d. Free or Nominal Rate Distribution (By Mail and Outside the Mail)	(1)	Free or Nominal Rate Outside-County Copies included on PS Form 3541	13	11
	(2)	Free or Nominal Rate In-County Copies Included on PS Form 3541	0	0
	(3)	Free or Nominal Rate Copies Mailed at Other Classes Through the USPS (e.g., First-Class Mail)	0	0
	(4)	Free or Nominal Rate Distribution Outside the Mail (Carriers or other means)	0	0
e. Total Free or Nominal Rate Distribution (Sum of 15d (1), (2), (3) and (4))			13	11
f. Total Distribution (Sum of 15c and 15e)			86	81
g. Copies not Distributed (See Instructions to Publishers #4 (page #3))			16	17
h. Total (Sum of 15f and g)			102	98
i. Percent Paid (15c divided by 15f times 100)			84.88%	86.41%

* If you are claiming electronic copies, go to line 16 on page 3. If you are not claiming electronic copies, skip to line 17 on page 3.

16. Electronic Copy Circulation	Average No. Copies Each Issue During Preceding 12 Months	No. Copies of Single Issue Published Nearest to Filing Date
a. Paid Electronic Copies ▶		
b. Total Paid Print Copies (Line 15c) + Paid Electronic Copies (Line 16a) ▶		
c. Total Print Distribution (Line 15f) + Paid Electronic Copies (Line 16a) ▶		
d. Percent Paid (Both Print & Electronic Copies) (16b divided by 16c × 100) ▶		

☒ I certify that 50% of all my distributed copies (electronic and print) are paid above a nominal price.

17. Publication of Statement of Ownership
☒ If the publication is a general publication, publication of this statement is required. Will be printed
in the OCTOBER 2021 issue of this publication.
☐ Publication not required.

18. Signature and Title of Editor, Publisher, Business Manager, or Owner

Malathi Samayan - Distribution Controller

Malathi Samayan

Date 9/18/2021

I certify that all information furnished on this form is true and complete. I understand that anyone who furnishes false or misleading information on this form or who omits material or information requested on the form may be subject to criminal sanctions (including fines and imprisonment) and/or civil sanctions (including civil penalties).

PS Form 3526, July 2014 (Page 3 of 4) PRIVACY NOTICE: See our privacy policy on www.usps.com

Printed and bound by CPI Group (UK) Ltd, Croydon, CR0 4YY

03/10/2024

01040403-0016